LOW-FAT COOKBOOK

+

DETOX COOKBOOK

2 in 1

A Low Fat & Detox Cookbook with Over 100 Quick & Easy Recipes

Karen Ward

Sommario

LOW-FAT

COOKBOOK

A Low Fat Cookbook with Over 50 Quick & Easy Recipes

Karen Ward

All rights reserved.

Disclaimer

The information contained i is meant to serve as a comprehensive collection of strategies that the author of this eBook has done research about. Summaries, strategies, tips and tricks are only recommendation by the author, and reading this eBook will not guarantee that one's results will exactly mirror the author's results. The author of the eBook has made all reasonable effort to provide current and accurate information for the readers of the eBook. The author and it's associates will not be held liable for any unintentional error or omissions that may be found. The material in the eBook may include information by third parties. Third party materials comprise of opinions expressed by their owners. As such, the author of the eBook does not assume responsibility or liability for any third party material or opinions. Whether because of the progression of the internet, or the unforeseen changes in company policy and editorial submission guidelines, what is stated as fact at the time of this writing may become outdated or inapplicable later.

The eBook is copyright © 2021 with all rights reserved. It is illegal to redistribute, copy, or create derivative work from this eBook whole or in part. No parts of this report may be reproduced or retransmitted in any reproduced or retransmitted in any forms whatsoever without the writing expressed and signed permission from the author

INTRODUCTION

A low-fat diet reduces the amount of fat that is ingested through food, sometimes drastically. Depending on how extreme this diet or nutrition concept is implemented, a mere 30 grams of fat may be consumed per day.

With conventional wholefood nutrition according to the interpretation of the German Nutrition Society, the recommended value is more than twice as high (approx. 66 grams or 30 to 35 percent of the daily energy intake). By greatly reducing dietary fat, the pounds should drop and / or not sit back on the hips.

Even if there are no prohibited foods per se with this diet: With liver sausage, cream and French fries you have reached the daily limit for fat faster than you can say "far from full". Therefore, for a low-fat diet, mainly or exclusively foods with a low fat content should end up on the plate - preferably "good" fats such as those in fish and vegetable oils.

WHAT ARE THE BENEFITS OF A LOW-FAT DIET?

Fat provides vital (essential) fatty acids. The body also needs fat to be able to absorb certain vitamins (A, D, E, K) from food. Eliminating fat in your diet altogether would therefore not be a good idea.

In fact, especially in wealthy industrial nations, significantly more fat is consumed every day than is recommended by experts. One problem with this is that fat is particularly rich in energy - one gram of it contains 9.3 calories and thus twice as many as one gram of carbohydrates or protein. An increased intake of fat therefore promotes obesity. In addition, too many saturated fatty acids, such as those in butter, lard or chocolate, are said to increase the risk of cardiovascular diseases and even cancer. Eating low-fat diets could prevent both of these problems.

LOW FAT FOODS: TABLE FOR LEAN ALTERNATIVES

Most people should be aware that it is not healthy to stuff yourself into uncontrolled fat. Obvious sources of fat such as fat rims on meat and sausage or butter lakes in the frying pan are easy to avoid.

It becomes more difficult with hidden fats, such as those found in pastries or cheese. With the latter, the amount of fat is sometimes given as an absolute percentage, sometimes as "% FiTr.", I.e. the fat content in the dry matter that arises when the water is removed from the food .

For a low-fat diet you have to look carefully, because a cream quark with 11.4% fat sounds lower in fat than one with 40% FiTr .. Both products have the same fat content. Lists from nutrition experts (e.g. the DGE) help to integrate a low-fat diet into everyday life as easily as possible and to avoid tripping hazards. For example, here is an instead of a table (high-fat foods with low-fat alternatives):

High fat foods

Low fat alternatives

Butter

Cream cheese, herb quark, mustard, sour cream, tomato paste

French fries, fried potatoes, croquettes, potato pancakes

Jacket potatoes, baked potatoes or baked potatoes

Pork belly, sausage, goose, duck

Veal, venison, turkey, pork cutlet, -lende, chicken, duck breast without skin

Lyoner, mortadella, salami, liver sausage, black pudding, bacon

Cooked / smoked ham without a fat rim, low-fat sausages such as salmon ham, turkey breast, roast meats, aspic sausage

Fat-free alternatives to sausage or cheese or to combine with them

Tomato, cucumber, radish slices, lettuce on bread or even banana slices / thin apple wedges, strawberries

Fish sticks

Steamed, low-fat fish

Tuna, salmon, mackerel, herring

Steamed cod, saithe, haddock

Milk, yoghurt (3.5% fat)

Milk, yoghurt (1.5% fat)

Cream quark (11.4% fat = 40% FiTr.)

Quark (5.1% fat = 20% FiTr.)

Double cream cheese (31.5% fat)

Layered cheese (2.0% fat = 10% FiTr.)

Fat cheese (> 15% fat = 30% FiTr.)

Low-fat cheeses (max. 15% fat = max. 30% FiTr.)

Creme fraiche (40% fat)

Sour cream (10% fat)

Mascarpone (47.5% fat)

Grainy cream cheese (2.9% fat)

Fruit cake with short crust pastry

Fruit cake with yeast or sponge batter

Sponge cake, cream cake, chocolate chip cookies, shortbread, chocolate, bars

Low-fat sweets such as Russian bread, ladyfingers, dried fruits, gummy bears, fruit gums, mini chocolate kisses (attention: sugar!)

Nut nougat cream, chocolate slices

Grainy cream cheese with a little jam

Croissants

Pretzel croissants, whole meal rolls, yeast pastries

Nuts, potato chips

Salt sticks or pretzels

Ice cream

Fruit ice cream

Black olives (35.8% fat)

green olives (13.3% fat)

LOW-FAT DIET: HOW TO SAVE FAT IN THE HOUSEHOLD

In addition to exchanging ingredients, there are a few other tricks you can use to incorporate a low-fat diet into your everyday life:

Steaming, stewing and grilling are fat-saving cooking methods for a low-fat diet.

Cook in the Römertopf or with special stainless steel pots. Food can also be prepared without fat in coated pans or in the foil.

You can also save fat with a pump sprayer: fill in about half of the oil and water, shake it and spray it on the base of the cookware before frying. If you don't have a pump sprayer, you can grease the cookware with a brush - this also saves fat.

For a low-fat diet in cream sauces or casseroles, replace half of the cream with milk.

Let soups and sauces cool down and then scoop the fat off the surface.

Prepare sauces with a little oil, sour cream or milk.

Roast and vegetable stocks can be tied with pureed vegetables or grated raw potatoes for a low-fat diet.

Put parchment paper or foil on the baking sheet, then there is no need to grease.

Just add a small piece of butter and fresh herbs to vegetable dishes, and the eyes will soon eat too.

Tie cream dishes with gelatin.

LOW FAT DIET: HOW HEALTHY IS IT REALLY?

For a long time, nutrition experts have been convinced that a low-fat diet is the key to a slim figure and health. Butter, cream and red meat, on the other hand, were considered a danger to the heart, blood values and scales. However, more and more studies suggest that fat isn't actually as bad as it gets. In contrast to a reduced-fat nutrition plan, test subjects could, for example, stick to a Mediterranean menu with lots of vegetable oil and fish, were healthier and still did not get fat.

When comparing different studies on fat, American researchers found that there was no connection between the consumption of saturated fat and the risk of coronary heart disease. There was also no clear scientific evidence that low-fat diets prolong life. Only so-called trans fats , which are produced, among other things, during deep-frying and the partial hardening of vegetable fats (in french fries, chips, ready-made baked goods etc.), were classified as dangerous by the scientists.

Those who only or mainly eat low-fat or fat-free foods probably eat more consciously overall, but run the risk of getting too little of the "good fats". There is also a risk of a lack of fat-soluble vitamins, which our body needs fat to absorb.

Low-fat diet: the bottom line

A low-fat diet requires dealing with the foods that one intends to consume. As a result, one is likely to be more conscious of buying, cooking and eating.

For weight loss, however, it is not primarily where the calories come from that counts, but that you take in less of them per day than you use. Even more: (Essential) fats are necessary for general health, since without them the body cannot utilize certain nutrients and cannot carry out certain metabolic processes.

In summary, this means: a low-fat diet can be an effective means of weight control or one to compensate for fat indulgence. It is not advisable to do without dietary fat entirely.

ZUCCHINI SALAD

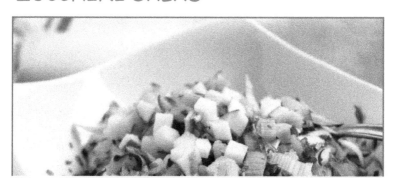

Serevings:2

INGREDIENTS

- 1 Pc zucchini
- 1 Pc Apple
- 2 Pc Spring onion
- 1 prize   salt
- 2 TbspMint, fresh

PREPARATION

Roughly grate the cleaned and washed zucchini in a bowl and season with salt. Let it steep a little and pour off the resulting water.

Then peel the apple and grate with the zucchini. Wash and clean the onion and cut into rings. Finally mix in the chopped mint into the salad.

ZUCCHINI DRESSING

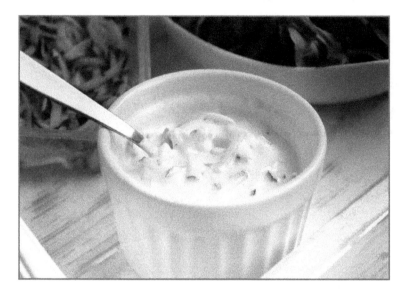

S

Serevings:2

INGREDIENTS

- 3 Tbsp   Sour cream
- 2 Tbsp   Mayonnaise, low fat
- 2 Tbsp   Zucchini, grated
- 2 Tbsp   Onion, grated
- 1 prize   salt

PREPARATION

Finely grate the washed zucchini and peeled onion in a bowl. Then mix in the mayonnaise and sour cream and season well with salt and pepper.

WATERMELON SALAD WITH FETA

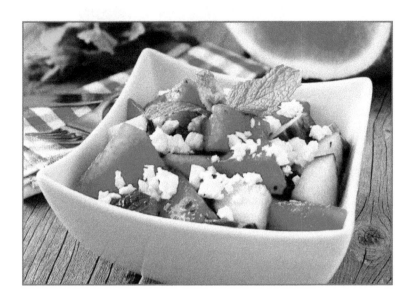

Serevings:4

INGREDIENTS

- 1   Pc Watermelon
- 1   Pc Cucumber
- 150   GFeta cheese
- 1   Federation Mint, fresh

for the dressing

- 2 Tbsp   honey
- 1 Pc   Lime, the juice of it
- 1 prize   salt

PREPARATION

For this fruity salad, first halve and quarter the watermelon, remove the pulp from the skin and then cut into cubes.

Roughly chop the feta, wash the mint leaves and cut into small pieces. Wash the cucumber, remove the stalk and cut into small pieces.

Then put the melon pieces together with the feta, pieces of cucumber and mint leaves in a bowl and mix well.

For the dressing, mix the honey with the lime juice and salt and pour over the salad.

WHOLE FOOD CASSEROLE WITH POTATOES AND TOMATOES

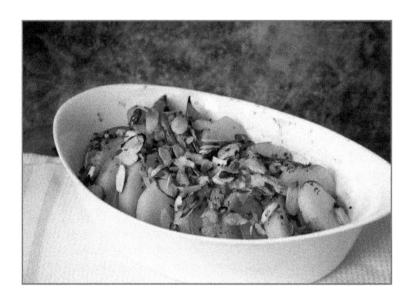

Serevings:4

INGREDIENTS

- 750 G   Potatoes, waxy
- 2   l   Water, for boiling the potatoes
- 1.5 TL Salt, for cooking the potatoes
- 750 G tomatoes
- 2 Tbsp   Gomasio, sesame salt
- 1 Pc onion
- 1 Pc clove of garlic
- 1 Tbsp   margarine
- 2 Tbsp   Basil, dried
- 100 G Flaked almonds

- 1 Tbsp   Margarine, for the mold

PREPARATION

First peel the potatoes, wash them, cut them into slices, cook them in a saucepan with salted water for about 10 minutes and then drain the water.

In the meantime, wash the tomatoes, remove the buds and cut into slices about the same thickness as the potato slices.

Then peel the onion and garlic and cut into fine cubes.

Melt the margarine (or butter) in a pan and sauté the onion and garlic pieces over low heat for about 5 minutes.

Now grease a casserole dish with margarine and put in the tomato and potato slices in alternating layers; Sprinkle each layer with a little Gomasio. Now preheat the oven to 220 ° C top and bottom heat.

Then distribute the steamed pieces of onion and garlic bellies as well as the basil and flaked almonds evenly over the casserole.

Finally, bake the whole casserole with potatoes and tomatoes in the preheated oven for about 10 minutes.

WHOLE GRAIN STICKS

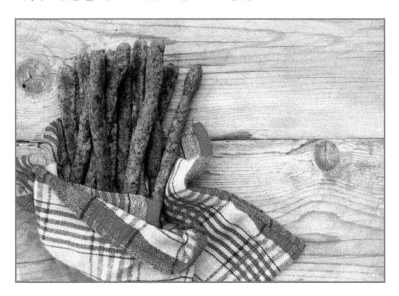

S

Serevings:1

INGREDIENTS

- 320 G   Whole wheat flour
- 0.5 Pk baking powder
- 1 TL salt
- 140 G lowfat quark
- 7 Tbsp   Sunflower oil
- 5 Tbsp   milk
- 3 Tbsp   Milk for brushing

PREPARATION

Put whole wheat flour, baking powder and salt in a bowl, mix and mix with the quark, oil and milk to a smooth dough.

Now shape the dough into a roll and cut 40 equal pieces with a knife. Shape each piece of dough into a thin, long stick.

Place these on a baking sheet lined with baking paper and brush with milk.

The whole grain Stangerl in a preheated oven at 180 ° C (hot air) (only one plate) Bake about 20 minutes.

VEGETARIAN POINTED CABBAGE STEW

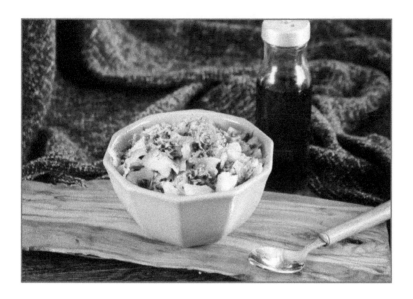

Serevings:4

INGREDIENTS

- 1 kg cabbage
- 300 G   Potatoes, mostly waxy, small
- 2 Pc Onions
- 1 Stg Leeks, leeks
- 2 Tbsp   Rapeseed oil, for the pot
- 1 l   Vegetable broth, unsalted

For spices

- 2   Pc Garlic cloves
- 2 Tbsp   sea-salt
- 0.5 TL   Pepper, white, freshly ground

- 0.5 TL   Nutmeg, freshly grated
- 1 TL Fennel seeds
- 1 TL   Cumin seeds
- 1 Pc   Cinnamon stick, small
- 1 Pc   Bay leaf
- 1 prize   Sea salt, to taste

PREPARATION

Peel and finely dice the onions and garlic. Clean the leek, slit lengthways, wash thoroughly and dice.

Then quarter the pointed cabbage lengthways, remove the stalk and cut the cabbage into bite-sized pieces. Peel and wash the potatoes and cut into 2 cm cubes.

Heat the rapeseed oil in a large saucepan and sweat the onion and garlic cubes in it for about 3-4 minutes.

Then add the pointed cabbage, potatoes and leek. Then season with sea salt, pepper and nutmeg and add the fennel seeds, caraway seeds, cinnamon stick and bay leaf and sauté briefly.

Now pour in the vegetable stock and simmer the vegetarian pointed cabbage stew over low heat for about 25 minutes.

Finally fish out the bay leaf and the cinnamon stick. Season the stew with sea salt again and serve hot.

VEGETARIAN SOLYANKA

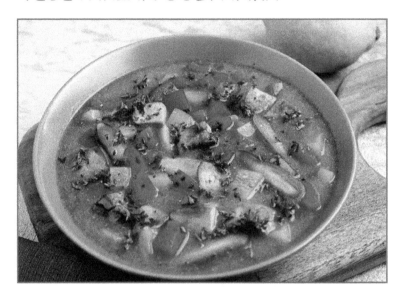

S

Serevings:2

INGREDIENTS

- 200 G   Smoked tofu
- 2 Pc Paprika, red and yellow
- 2 Pc   Onions
- 200 G   Tomato paste
- 6   Pc gherkins
- 150 ml   Pickle water
- 800 ml   Vegetable broth, hot
- 1 TL   Cane sugar, brown sugar
- 1 TL Lemon juice
- 1   TL Paprika powder, hot as rose

- 1 prize   Pepper, black, ground
- 125 ml   Whipped cream or soy cream
- 1 prize   salt
- 2 Tbsp   Parsley, chopped
- 5 Tbsp   Rapeseed oil

PREPARATION

Halve, core, wash the peppers and cut into small cubes. Also cut the smoked tofu into cubes.

Peel the onions and chop them into fine pieces. Cut the pickles into small pieces.

Next, heat the rapeseed oil in a saucepan and fry the tofu cubes in it for about 6-8 minutes until crispy and brown.

Then add the onion and pepper cubes to the tofu and fry for about 5 minutes. Add 140 grams of the tomato paste and roast for 1 minute.

Now pour in the vegetable broth, add the pickled cucumbers, the pickled cucumber water and the remaining tomato paste and bring to the boil for 1 minute.

Then season the vegetarian solyanka with salt, pepper, cane sugar and paprika powder and simmer at a low temperature for about 45-55 minutes.

Season the finished soup with whipped cream and lemon juice and add the chopped parsley just before serving.

VEGAN CHILLI

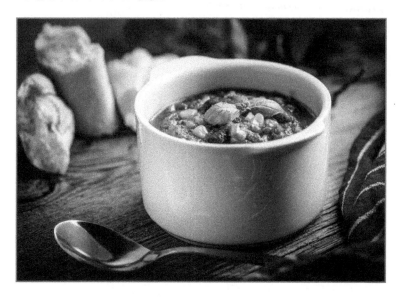

S

Serevings:4

INGREDIENTS

- 120 G Soy granules
- 500 ml   Vegetable broth, hot
- 3 Tbsp   Rapeseed oil
- 2 Pc Onions
- 0.5 TL   Paprika powder, hot
- 0.5 TL   Chilli flakes
- 1 Pc   clove of garlic
- 50 G Tomato paste
- 1 Can Tomatoes, á 400 g
- 250 G Kidney beans

- 1 Can Corn, á 400 g
- 1 TL salt
- 1 TL sugar
- 0.5 TL   Pepper, black, ground

PREPARATION

First heat the vegetable stock and soak the soy granules in it for about 8-10 minutes. Then pour into a sieve, collect the broth and allow the granules to drain well.

Meanwhile, peel and finely dice the onion and garlic. Heat the oil in a shallow saucepan and fry the soy granules with the onion cubes for about 5 minutes.

Then stir in the tomato paste and roast for 1 minute. Stir in garlic, paprika and chilli flakes.

Now drain the beans and corn and add with the tomatoes and the broth and simmer the vegan chilli over low heat for about 20-25 minutes.

Finally, season with salt, pepper and sugar, bring to the boil for 1 minute and serve.

VEGAN TOMATO DIP

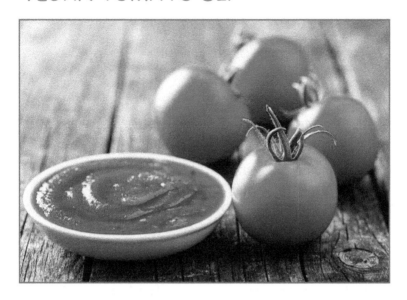

S

Serevings:8

INGREDIENTS

- 15 Tbsp   Tomato paste
- 15 Tbsp   Apple Cider Vinegar
- 250 G sugar
- 1 prize   salt
- 1 prize   pepper

PREPARATION

First take a small saucepan, add tomato paste, vinegar and sugar
and bring to the boil while stirring on a medium heat.

Then let everything cool down, season with salt and pepper and serve in a bowl.

VEGAN MANGO LASSI

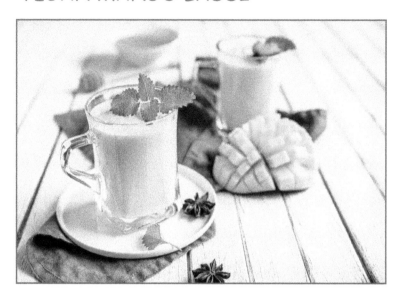

S

Serevings:2

- **INGREDIENTS**
- 1 Pc   ripe mango
- 300 G Lupine yogurt
- 150 ml   water
- 1 Tbsp   Agave syrup

PREPARATION

Peel the ripe mango, remove the pulp from the stone and then cut into large pieces.

Put the mango pieces together with the lupine yogurt, water and agave syrup in a blender and puree them finely.

The vegan mango lassi stuffed as desired with ice cubes into glasses and garnish with fresh herbs.

VEGAN STOCK POT

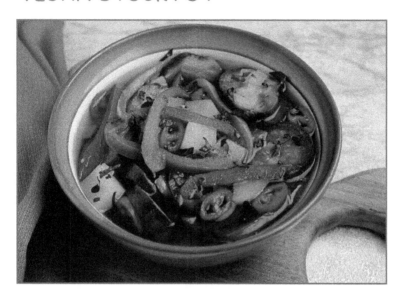

s

Serevings:4

INGREDIENTS

- 4 Pc Eggplant
- 2 Pc Chili peppers, red
- 4 Pc clove of garlic
- 4   Pc Bay leaf
- 4 Pc Paprika, colorful
- 1 Pc   onion
- 750 ml   Vegetable broth
- 2 Tbsp   olive oil
- 1 prize   salt
- 1 prize   Pepper from the grinder

- 1 prize   Paprika powder, hot as rose
- 300 G Potatoes

PREPARATION

First peel the onion and the garlic cloves and chop them into fine pieces. Then wash the eggplants and cut them into slices. Halve, core, wash and cut the bell pepper into strips.

Core, wash and cut the chilli peppers into small pieces. Peel the potatoes and cut into small cubes.

Now heat the olive oil in a saucepan over a medium flame and roast the onion and garlic cubes in it.

Then add the aubergine slices, paprika strips and the chilli pieces and also sauté briefly.

Now add the bay leaves and the potato cubes, pour in the vegetable stock and cook on a low heat for about 25 minutes.

Depending on your taste, season the vegan vegetable pot with salt, pepper and paprika powder and serve.

VEGAN FROZEN YOGURT

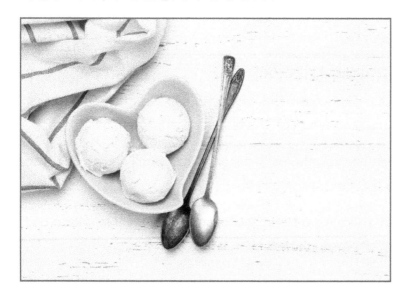

S

Serevings:4

INGREDIENTS

- 6 Tbsp   Maple syrup
- 6 Tbsp   Oat cuisine
- 400 G vegan yogurt (of your choice)
- 4 Tbsp   Oat drink

PREPARATION

To start, add the vegan yogurt, oat drink, maple syrup and coconut milk to the blender.

Mix everything well for one minute and then put in the ice cream maker for 40 minutes.

Finally, put the ice in a freezer and let it set in the freezer for at least 20 minutes.

VEGAN CREAM CHEESE MADE FROM CASHEW NUTS

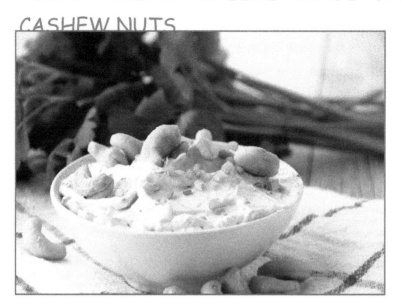

Serevings:5

INGREDIENTS

- 250 G   Cashew nuts, natural
- 2 Tbsp   Yeast flakes (from Rapunzel)
- 4 Tbsp   Apple Cider Vinegar
- 2 Tbsp   Lemon juice, from the bottle or straight
- 1 prize   salt and pepper
- 0.5 Federation   Chives, fresh

PREPARATION

To start, put the cashews in a large bowl and fill it with enough water to cover the kernels. Now let the whole thing soak overnight.

Then drain the cashew nuts and blend them together with yeast flakes, apple cider vinegar, lemon juice, water, salt and pepper in a blender for about a minute.

Meanwhile wash, dry and finely chop the chives. Then mix the mixer mass with the chives in a bowl, season the whole thing with salt and pepper again and the vegan cream cheese made from cashew nuts is ready .

VEGAN MUSHROOM SPREAD

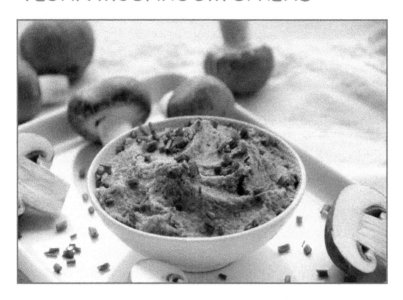

S

Serevings:4

INGREDIENTS

- 200 G Mushrooms
- 2 Pc Onions
- 100 ml   Soy cream
- 0.25 TL   salt
- 0.25 TL   pepper
- 2 Tbsp   Chives, chopped
- 2 Tbsp   Yeast flakes
- 1 Tbsp   Lemon juice
- 1 shot olive oil
- 1 Tbsp Almond butter

PREPARATION

To start, heat the olive oil in a pan, clean the mushrooms, cut into thin slices and fry in the pan with the olive oil for about 10 minutes until all the liquid has evaporated.

Meanwhile, peel the onions, cut into cubes and place in a bowl with soy cream, almond butter and lemon juice.

Then take the mushrooms out of the pan, add them to the bowl and add the yeast flakes, salt, pepper and chives.

Finally, put all the ingredients in a blender and mix the vegan mushroom spread to a creamy mass

VEGAN SPREAD WITH BEETROOT AND HORSERADISH

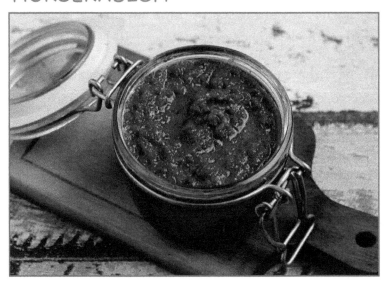

Serevings:8

INGREDIENTS

- 100 G Sweet lupins, ground
- 2 Tbsp   Tahini (sesame mushroom)
- 4 Tbsp   olive oil
- 1 TL Lemon juice
- 1 prize   salt
- 1 prize   pepper
- 1 Kn Beetroot, pre-cooked
- 1 TL Cream horseradish

PREPARATION

First prepare the crushed sweet lupins according to the instructions on the packet.

Then let the lupins cool down a little and finely puree them with tahini, olive oil and lemon juice. Then season with salt and pepper.

Peel the beetroot, cut into large pieces, add to the lupins together with the horseradish and puree again.

Finally , fill the vegan spread with beetroot and horseradish into a clean, sealable glass and store in the refrigerator.

VEGAN OVERNIGHT OATS WITH STRAWBERRIES

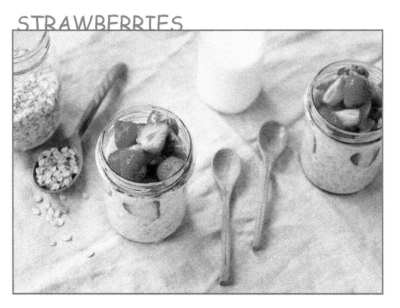

Serevings:4

INGREDIENTS

- 200 G   oatmeal
- 500 ml   Almond milk
- 500 G Strawberries
- 4 TL honey

PREPARATION

Mix the oat flakes with almond milk the evening before and leave to swell overnight in the refrigerator.

The next morning, divide the overnight oats into four glasses. Wash, dry and quarter fresh strawberries.

Fold 3/4 of the mixture from the strawberries into the overnight oats and use 1/4 for decoration.

Finally, drizzle the overnight oats with honey if desired.

VEGAN MOUSSAKA

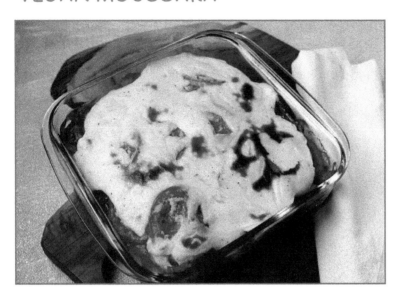

S

Serevings:4

INGREDIENTS

- 300 G   Potatoes, waxy
- 400 G aubergine
- 300 G zucchini
- 2 Pc Tomatoes, great
- 0.5 TL   Salt, for the cooking water
- 1 Tbsp   Olive oil, for the shape
- 1 prize   salt
- for the tomato sauce
- 2 Pc Garlic cloves
- 2 Pc Shallots

- 3 Tbsp   olive oil
- 2 Tbsp   Tomato paste
- 400 G Tomatoes, chopped, can
- 1 prize   sugar
- 400 ml   Vegetable broth, hot
- 2 TL   Thyme leaves, chopped
- 1 TL   Paprika powder, hot
- 1 prize   Ground cinnamon
- 0.5 TL   salt
- 1 prize   Pepper, black, ground

for the bechamel sauce

- 50 G Flour
- 50 G Vegetable margarine
- 350 ml   Soy drink
- 1 prize   salt
- 1 prize   Nutmeg, grated
- 1 prize   Pepper, white, ground

PREPARATION

First peel, wash and thinly slice the potatoes. Wash and clean the aubergine and zucchini, cut into thin slices and sprinkle with salt.

Then wash the tomatoes, remove the stem and cut into slices.

Bring the water with a little salt to a boil in a saucepan, add the potato slices and cook over a medium heat for about 8 minutes. Then drain and drain well.

For the tomato sauce, peel off the shallots and garlic and chop finely.

Heat the olive oil in a pan, sauté the garlic and shallots for about 2 minutes until translucent and stir in the tomato paste.

Then deglaze with the vegetable stock, add the canned tomatoes and bring to the boil for 1 minute. Then reduce the heat, season with sugar, thyme, cinnamon, paprika powder, salt and pepper and simmer for about 5 minutes.

Meanwhile, preheat the oven to 180 ° C (fan oven 160 ° C) and grease a baking dish with olive oil.

Now layer half of the aubergine, potato and zucchini slices in the mold and pour the tomato sauce over them. Layer the remaining vegetable slices and cover with the remaining sauce. Finally, put the tomato slices on top.

For the bechamel sauce, melt the margarine in a saucepan, add the flour, stirring constantly, and sweat for about 2 minutes.

Then pour in the soy drink and cook for about 3-4 minutes, stirring, until the sauce is thick and smooth. Finally, season the sauce with salt, pepper and nutmeg.

Now pour the béchamel sauce over the vegan moussaka and bake on the middle rack in the preheated oven for about 45 minutes.

VEGAN LENTIL SOUP

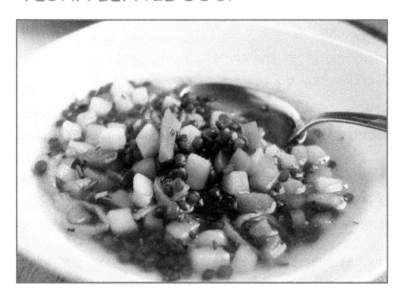

S

Serevings:4

INGREDIENTS

- 250 G Lentils, brown
- 1 Stg leek
- 2 Pc Carrots
- 1 Pc onion
- 2 l Vegetable broth, hot
- 3 Pc Potatoes, waxy
- 1 Tbsp   Vegetable oil
- 1 prize   salt
- 1 prize Pepper, black, ground
- 1 prize   sugar

- 2 Tbsp   Parsley, chopped

PREPARATION

First peel the potatoes and carrots, wash them and cut them into small cubes. Peel the onion and finely chop.

Then clean the leek, wash it thoroughly and cut it into fine rings. Put the lentils in a colander, rinse under cold water and drain.

Heat the oil in a stock pot and sauté the lentils, carrots, onions and leeks in it for about 1 minute. Pour in the vegetable stock and bring to the boil.

As soon as the soup boils, reduce the temperature and cover and let the soup simmer gently for about 15 minutes.

Next, add the potato cubes to the soup and simmer for another 15 minutes. Finally, season with salt, pepper and sugar.

Fill the finished vegan lentil soup into soup bowls, sprinkle with the parsley and enjoy.

VEGAN PUMPKIN SOUP

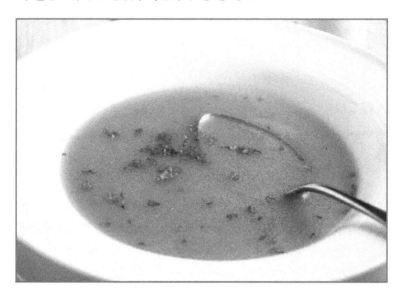

S

Serevings:4

INGREDIENTS

- 1   kg Hokkaido pumpkin
- 300 gl   sweet potato
- 500 ml   Vegetable broth, hot
- 1 Can Coconut milk, unsweetened, á 400 ml
- 1 Pc   onion
- 2 Pc Garlic cloves
- 1 Tbsp   Coconut oil
- 15 G Ginger, fresh
- 1 TL Paprika powder, noble sweet
- 0.5 TL   turmeric

- 0.5 TL   Coriander, ground
- 1 prize   Pepper, black, freshly ground
- 1 prize   salt
- 2 Tbsp   Olive oil, for brushing
- 2 Tbsp   Parsley, chopped

PREPARATION

First preheat the oven to 200 ° C top / bottom heat and line a baking sheet with baking paper.

Then wash the sweet potato and prick it several times with a fork. Wash the pumpkin, cut in half and scrape out the seeds including the fibers. Cut the pumpkin into wedges.

Place the potato and pumpkin wedges on the baking sheet and brush with olive oil. Roast in the preheated oven on the middle rack for about 40-45 minutes. Then take it out of the oven, let it cool down for 10 minutes, peel and dice the sweet potatoes.

Peel and finely chop the onion and garlic. Peel the ginger and also finely chop it. Heat the oil in a stock pot over medium heat and sweat the onion and garlic cubes in it for about 2 minutes.

Now add the ginger and fry for 1 minute. Add the potatoes, pumpkin, paprika powder, turmeric and coriander, pour in the coconut milk and the broth and bring everything to a boil. Bring the contents of the pot to the boil for 1 minute, reduce the temperature and simmer gently for another 10 minutes.

Purée finely with the help of a cutting stick. If the soup is still too thick, stir in a little broth. Season to taste with salt and pepper.

The vegan pumpkin soup into preheated soup bowls fill, sprinkle with parsley and enjoy.

VEGAN GUACAMOLE

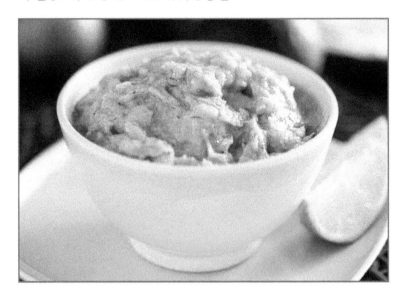

S

Serevings:4

INGREDIENTS

- 2   Pc Avocados
- 2   Pc Lime, the juice
- 3   Pc clove of garlic
- 1   TL Chili powder, mild
- 1 prize   salt
- 1 prize   Pepper from the grinder

PREPARATION

Halve the avocados, remove the stone and puree the pulp with the lime juice, squeezed garlic and chili powder using a blender.

Season to taste with salt and pepper before serving.

VEGAN BROCCOLI CREAM SOUP WITH WHITE BEANS

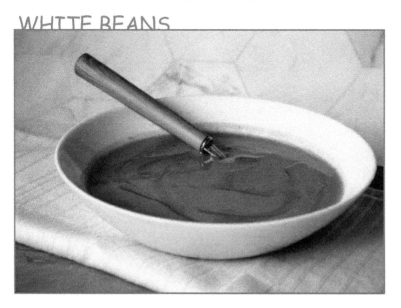

Serevings:4

INGREDIENTS

- 1 kpf broccoli
- 400 G   white beans, pre-cooked
- 1 Stg leek
- 2 Pc Garlic cloves
- 800 ml   Vegetable broth
- 1 TL salt
- 0.5 TL   Pepper, freshly ground
- 0.5 TL   Paprika powder

PREPARATION

First clean the leek, wash it well and cut it into fine rings. Peel and dice the garlic. Clean the broccoli, cut into florets and wash.

Then fry the leek and garlic with a dash of vegetable stock in a large saucepan on a medium heat until translucent.

Then add the broccoli florets and cook for about 5 minutes.

Then add the white beans and vegetable stock, bring to the boil, season with salt, pepper and paprika and simmer for about 10 minutes until the broccoli is cooked through.

Finally, mix the soup with a hand blender until creamy and add a little more seasoning if necessary

VANILLA SAUCE WITHOUT SUGAR

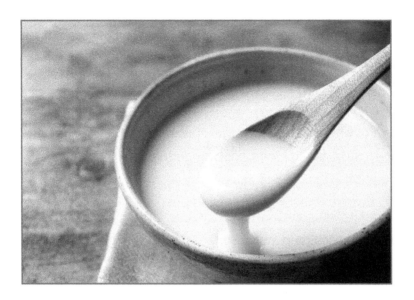

Servings:4

INGREDIENTS

- 500 ml   milk
- 1.5Tbsp   food starch
- 1 Pc egg yolk
- 1 Pc   Vanilla pod
- 3 Tr Stevia, liquid sweetener to taste

PREPARATION

First put the cornstarch in a bowl. Then add the egg yolk to the cornstarch and beat with the whisk of a hand mixer for about 2 minutes.

Then add about 6-7 tablespoons of the milk and beat for another 3-4 minutes.

Next, slit open the vanilla pod, scrape out the pulp and add to the egg milk. Mix with the whisk for another 1 minute.

Now heat the rest of the milk in a saucepan, bring to the boil for 1 minute and then remove from the stove. Stir the vanilla starch milk into the hot milk, stir in thoroughly and place back on the stove.

The vanilla sauce without sugar can, stirring once again boil 1 minute and make sure that they do not burn. Finally - depending on your taste - stir in 2-3 drops of liquid sweetness and let the sauce cool down.

BAKED FENNEL WITH MOZZARELLA

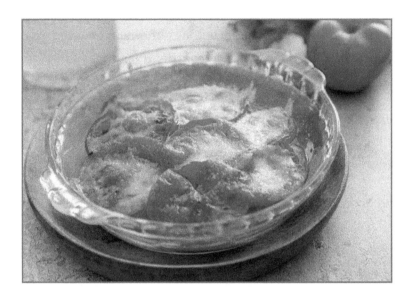

Serevings:4

INGREDIENTS

- 4 Kn fennel
- 2 Pc tomatoes
- 4 Tbsp   Lemon juice
- 250 G Mozzarella
- 1 Pc   Bay leaf
- 1 between   rosemary
- 1 between   thyme
- 150 ml   White wine, dry
- 350 ml   Vegetable broth
- 1 prize   salt
- 1 prize   Ground pepper
- 2 Tbsp   Oil, for greasing

PREPARATION

First preheat the oven to 200 ° C top and bottom heat / 180 ° C convection and grease a casserole dish with a little oil.

Then wash and dry the fennel, cut off the hard ends and cut into fine strips.

Now put the wine together with the vegetable stock in a saucepan, bring everything to a boil and simmer over medium heat for 4-6 minutes.

In the meantime, wash, dry and finely chop the rosemary and thyme.

Then add the chopped herbs together with the bay leaf and a pinch of salt and pepper to the pot.

Then add the fennel to the pot and cook it for 4-6 minutes.

Meanwhile, drain the mozzarella and cut into slices.

Then wash the tomatoes, dry them and also cut them into thin slices.

In the next step, drain the fennel, drain well, place in the baking dish and drizzle with the lemon juice.

Finally, put the tomatoes and mozzarella in the baking dish and bake the fennel in the oven for around 10 minutes.

FANTASTICALLY SWEET YEAST DOUGH

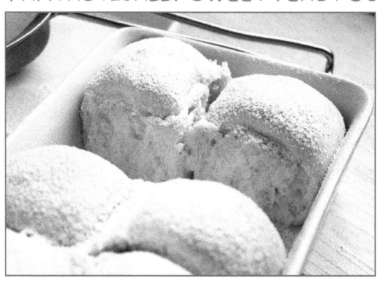

Serevings:1

- **INGREDIENTS**
- 500 G Spelled flour type 630
- 250 ml   Soy drink
- 120 G Raw cane sugar
- 1 prize   salt
- 2 Tbsp   Sunflower oil
- 42 G Fresh yeast

PREPARATION

First crumble the yeast cube in a dough bowl, add the soy drink and 2 tablespoons of raw cane sugar, stir briefly and let rest for about 10 minutes.

Then add the flour, salt, sunflower oil and the remaining raw cane sugar and knead everything thoroughly for several minutes, ideally with a food processor or a slow hand mixer with a dough hook.

As soon as a smooth, even batter has formed, moisten a clean tea towel and place it over the bowl. Finally, put it in a warm place for about four hours so that the dough can rise in peace.

Depending on the additional recipe for which the wonderfully sweet yeast dough is used, the baking time is around 30 minutes at 180 ° C (convection).

TOMATOSOUP

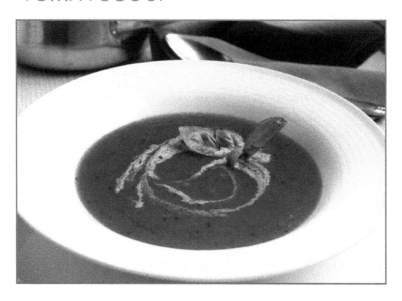

S

Serevings:4

INGREDIENTS

- 1 l   light bone broth
- 500 G tomatoes
- 60 G butter
- 50 G Root system
- 1 Pc onion
- 40 G Flour
- 1 shot vinegar
- 1 TL sugar
- 0.5 TL   Peppercorns
- 1 TL salt

- 2 Pc garlic

PREPARATION

Peel or clean the roots, peel the onion and garlic and cut the ingredients into small pieces. Roast some peppercorns with a little butter.

Lightly sweat the whole thing with a little flour and pour 1 liter of bone soup on top.

Then tear up the skinned tomatoes and stir into the broth with tomato paste.

The soup is cooked for another 25 minutes with salt, vinegar and sugar.

Finally, finely strain the tomato soup using a sieve.

TOMATO SOUP WITHOUT SUGAR

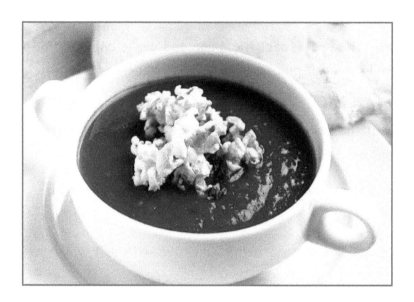

Serevings:2

INGREDIENTS

- 100 GMicrowave popcorn, lightly salted
- 3 Pc Carrots
- 10 Pc Cocktail tomatoes, red
- 0.5 l Vegetable broth
- 0.5 Pc onion
- 1 prize   salt
- 1 prize   Pepper, black, ground

PREPARATION

First let the popcorn puff up in the microwave for about 3-4 minutes, then remove it and set it aside.

Peel, wash and grate the carrots on a sharp grater. Bring the vegetable stock to a boil in a saucepan, add the carrots and cook for about 12-15 minutes until soft.

Meanwhile, wash the tomatoes and cut them in half. Peel the onions and cut into fine wedges. Add tomatoes and onions to the soup and simmer for another 30 minutes over low heat.

Finally puree everything finely with a cutting stick and bring to the boil for another 1 minute.

The tomato soup without sugar to taste with salt and pepper and place in a warm plate. Add the popcorn to the soup as a topping and serve.

TOMATO SOUP WITH RICE

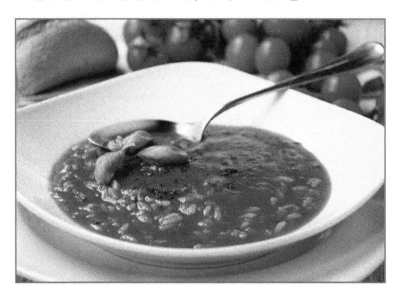

S

Serevings:4

INGREDIENTS

- 2 Pc onion
- 2 Tbsp Olive oil, for the pot
- 150 G Long grain rice
- 1 l Tomato juice
- 1 TL salt
- 1 prize Pepper White
- 0.5 TL sugar
- 3 TbspParsley, freshly chopped
- 0.5 TL Marjoram, finely chopped

PREPARATION

For the tomato soup with rice, first peel and finely chop the onions. Then heat the oil in a saucepan and sauté the onion pieces in it.

Then wash the rice, add to the onions and stir-fry for 1-2 minutes.

Then pour in the tomato juice, sprinkle in the marjoram, salt and pepper, bring to the boil and simmer covered over low heat for about 15-20 minutes until the rice is cooked.

Finally, season the soup again with salt, pepper and sugar, sprinkle with chopped parsley and serve garnished with a basil leaf.

TOMATO SOUP WITH PEARL BARLEY

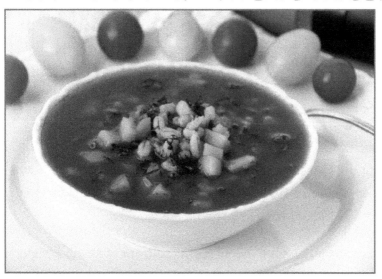

Serevings:2

INGREDIENTS

- 1 Can Tomatoes, á 800 g
- 1 Federation Soup greens (celery, carrots, leek)
- 1 Pc onion
- 1 Pc clove of garlic
- 75 G Pearl barley
- 6 Pc Sage leaves
- 1 Tbsp   olive oil
- 750 ml   Vegetable broth
- 6 Tbsp   Creme fraiche Cheese
- 4 Tbsp   Parmesan, freshly grated

- 1 prize   salt
- 1 prize   Pepper, black, freshly ground

PREPARATION

First peel the carrots and celery, then wash and dice. Clean the leek, wash it thoroughly and also cut it into small cubes.

Peel the onion and garlic and dice very finely. Then wash the sage and cut it into fine strips.

Next, heat the olive oil in a soup pot and fry the diced vegetables, onion and garlic in it for about 3-4 minutes. Then add the sage leaves and the pearl barley and fry for 2-3 minutes.

Now add the stock and the juice of the canned tomatoes. Roughly chop the canned tomatoes and add them as well.

The tomato soup with pearl barley can then simmer for about 30 minutes at medium temperature.

Finally stir in the crème fraîche and the grated Parmesan cheese into the soup, season with salt and pepper and serve hot.

TOMATO RAGOUT WITH EGGPLANT

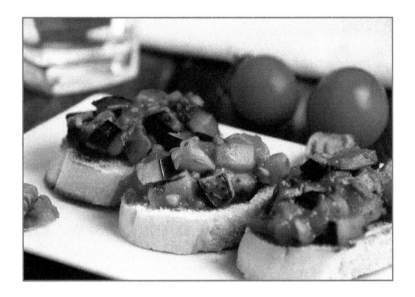

Serevings:4

INGREDIENTS

- 2 Pc Eggplant, medium size
- 4 Pc Tomatoes, great
- 2 Pc Garlic cloves
- 2 Tbsp Basil, chopped
- 1 prize salt
- 1 TL olive oil
- 1 prize pepper

PREPARATION

Peel the garlic cloves, press them through a garlic press and sauté lightly in a pan with oil.

Remove the stalk from the eggplant, peel, cut into small cubes and mix in the pan with the garlic.

Then wash the tomatoes, cut them into small pieces and also mix in the pan. Fry the vegetables in the pan for about 6-8 minutes - stirring constantly.

Then season with salt, pepper and fresh basil to taste and serve with white bread.

TOMATOES FILLED WITH SPINACH

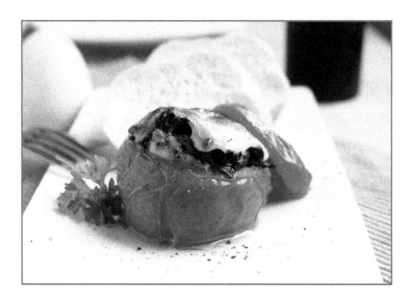

Serevings:4

INGREDIENTS

- 4 Pc Beefsteak tomatoes
- 1 Pc onion
- 2 Pc Garlic cloves
- 175 G Spinach leaves
- 2 Tbsp   olive oil
- 60 G Sheep cheese
- 3 Tbsp   Gratin cheese (grated)
- 1 prize   salt and pepper
- 1 prize   Nutmeg (ground)

PREPARATION

Cut off a lid from the washed tomatoes, scrape out the pulp with a spoon and place the tomatoes in an oiled baking dish.

Wash and drain the spinach.

Peel onion and garlic, chop finely and sauté in hot olive oil until translucent. Then add the spinach, stew until al dente and mix with the sheep's cheese.

Then season the spinach mixture with nutmeg, salt and pepper, pour into the tomatoes, sprinkle the grated cheese on top and place the tomatoes filled with spinach in the preheated oven (180 ° C) for 10 minutes.

TOMATOES WRAPPED IN CUCUMBER

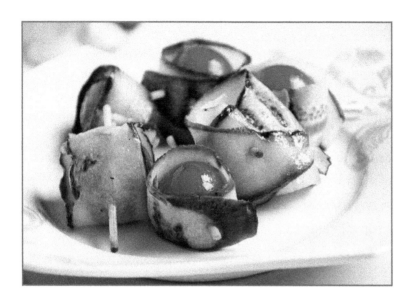

Serevings:2

INGREDIENTS

- 8 Pc Cocktail tomatoes
- 1 shot olive oil
- 2 Pc Cucumbers
- 1 prize Spices (salt, pepper, etc.)

PREPARATION

Remove the ends of the cucumber and cut lengthways into thin slices. Place the cucumber slices on the work surface. Put one tomato on each and wrap it tightly.

So that the whole thing holds together, it is fixed with toothpicks. Just season, brush with olive oil and place on the hot grill (5-7 min.)

COLD TOMATO BOWL

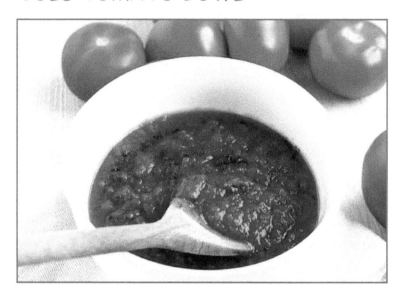

S

Serevings:4

INGREDIENTS

- 1   kg Tomatoes, canned, diced
- 4   Pc clove of garlic
- 3   between   basil
- 600 ml   Vegetable broth
- 1 Pc Orange, juice
- 1 prize   salt

PREPARATION

At the beginning peel and finely chop the garlic, also finely chop the washed basil.

Now bring the tomatoes, garlic, orange juice, basil and broth to the boil in a large saucepan and simmer for a few minutes over low heat.

Then puree the soup with the blender, add salt to taste and cover and chill for at least 4 hours.

TOMATO AND CUCUMBER STICKS

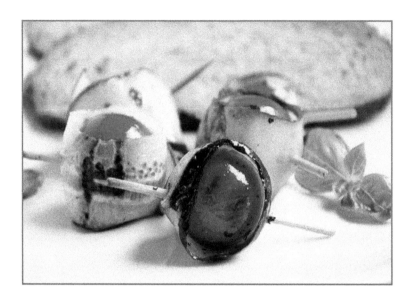

Serevings:2

INGREDIENTS

- 8 Pc Cherry tomatoes
- 1 prize   salt
- 1 Pc Cucumber
- 1 prize   Pepper (freshly ground)
- 1 shot olive oil
- 8 Pc Toothpick (to fix)

PREPARATION

Wash the cucumber and cut lengthways into wafer-thin slices
with a peeler.

Then place the cucumber slices on the worktop and season with salt and pepper. Now place the washed tomatoes on one of the ends, roll up tightly and fix with a toothpick.

Then brush with olive oil, place on the hot grill (or oven / grill) and grill for about 5 minutes.

THAI SWEET AND SOUR SAUCE

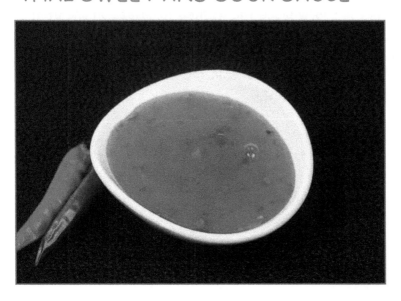

S

Serevings:4

INGREDIENTS

- 1 Pc red peppers, great
- 2 Pc Garlic cloves
- 1 Pc Chilli pepper
- 5 Tbsp   Rice vinegar
- 10Tbsp   sugar
- 250 ml   water

PREPARATION

In the first step, wash the peppers, cut in half, core and cut into small pieces, do the same with the chilli pepper.

Then peel the garlic, chop it roughly and put it in the blender along with the pieces of pepper, chilli pieces, vinegar and water. Then puree the whole thing for about a minute and then pour it into a small saucepan.

Now add sugar, stir in and simmer on low heat while stirring until the sauce thickens.

Then let it cool down and serve the finished Thai sweet and sour sauce in a bowl or over a dish.

SWEET POTATOES WITH COTTAGE CHEESE

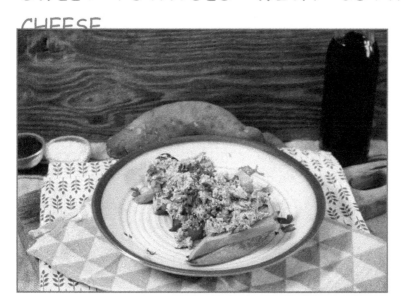

Serevings: 3

INGREDIENTS

- 2 Pc Sweet potatoes
- 2 Pc Carrots
- 3 Tbsp   Basil leaves
- 200 G Cottage cheese, cream cheese
- 1 prize   salt
- 1 prize   Paprika powder, noble sweet
- 1 prize   Ground pepper
- 3 Tbsp   Parsley, fresh

PREPARATION

First preheat the oven to 200 ° C top and bottom heat / 180 ° C circulating air.

In the meantime, wash and peel the sweet potatoes, cut into 6 equal slices or pieces, place on a baking sheet and bake in the oven for about 10 minutes.

In the meantime, wash and peel the carrots and grate them finely in a bowl with a kitchen grater.

Then wash the basil, shake it dry and finely chop it with a knife.

Then add the cottage cheese to the bowl and mix with salt, pepper, paprika and basil.

Now wash, dry and finely chop the parsley.

Finally, remove the sweet potatoes from the oven, brush with the cottage cheese and garnish with the parsley.

SWEET POTATO SALAD WITH SPINACH

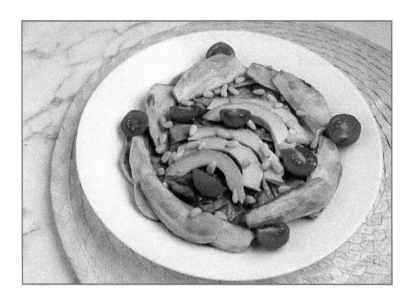

Serevings:4

INGREDIENTS

- 4 Pc   Medium sized sweet potatoes
- 150   G   Spinach, young
- 16   Pc Cherry tomatoes
- 80   G Pine nuts
- 4 Tbsp   olive oil
- 1 prize   salt
- 1 prize pepper
- 1 Pc   avocado

for the dressing

- 3 Tbsp   Honey, liquid

- 3 Tbsp   Red wine vinegar
- 2 Tbsp   olive oil
- 1 prize   salt
- 1 prize   pepper

PREPARATION

First peel and wash the sweet potatoes and cut them into even, thin wedges.

Sort the spinach, wash it thoroughly and dry it. Wash the cherry tomatoes and cut in half.

Now roast the pine nuts in a coated pan without fat - stir constantly, then take them out of the pan and let them cool down.

Now heat 4 tablespoons of olive oil in a non-stick pan, fry the sweet potato wedges in it over a moderate heat for about 15 minutes and season with salt and pepper.

Then peel the avocado, remove the stone and cut into thin wedges.

Now put the honey, vinegar and olive oil in a bowl, whisk thoroughly with the blender and season with salt and pepper.

Finally, distribute the spinach and avocado in the middle of the plates, then decorate the sweet potatoes with the tomatoes, drizzle with the dressing and serve the sweet potato salad with spinach sprinkled with the pine nuts.

SWEET POTATO CURRY CHIPS

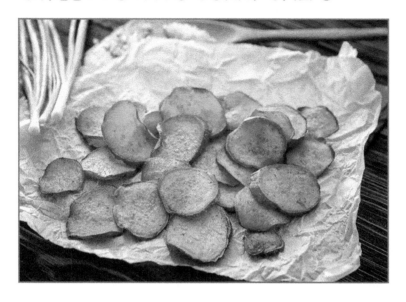

S

Serevings:2

INGREDIENTS

- 2   Pc Sweet potato, great
- 2 Tbsp   Oil, neutral
- 1 TL   curry
- 1 TL   salt
- 1 prize   Pepper, freshly ground

PREPARATION

Preheat the oven to 180 degrees and cover a baking sheet with baking paper.

Then wash the sweet potato thoroughly, cut it into thin slices or slice it and place it on the baking sheet.

Drizzle with oil and season with salt, pepper and curry, then bake the sweet potato curry chips in the hot oven for 20 minutes.

SWEET CARROTS

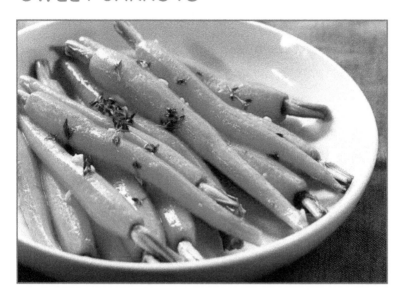

S

Serevings:4

INGREDIENTS

- 700 G Carrots, small
- 1 Tbsp   butter
- 3 Tbsphoney

PREPARATION

Wash and clean the carrots beforehand and cover with a little water and let them simmer over low heat.

Then heat the butter in a pan over medium heat, add the honey and the carrots and glaze the carrots while stirring constantly on a low heat. This takes about 1 to 2 minutes.

SWEET PUMPKIN RAW FOOD

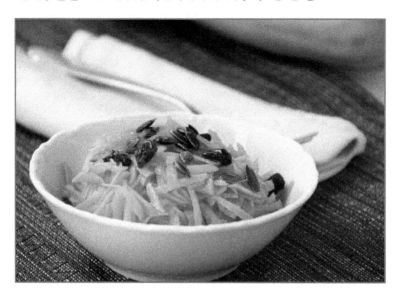

S

Serevings:3

INGREDIENTS

- 1 Pc Hokkaido pumpkin, small
- 1 prize   Vanilla, ground
- 1 prize   Organic cinnamon, Ceylon variety
- 2 Tbsp   Maple syrup (more if necessary)

PREPARATION

First, wash the pumpkin, cut it in half, remove the stone and grate it with a kitchen grater.

Then put the pulp in a nice bowl, stir in the vanilla, maple syrup and cinnamon and enjoy the finished, sweet raw pumpkin .

SWEET AND SOUR CHINESE CABBAGE SALAD

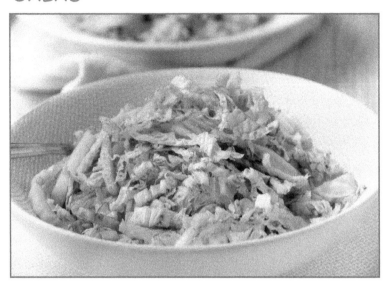

Serevings:2

INGREDIENTS

- 1 Pc Chinese cabbage

for the dressing

- 2 Tbsp   soy sauce
- 1 TL   honey
- 1 Tbsp   Rice vinegar
- 2 Pc   clove of garlic

PREPARATION

Remove the stalk from the Chinese cabbage, wash the leaves well and cut into strips. Then peel and finely chop the garlic.

Then stir in a dressing with the garlic, soy sauce, rice vinegar and honey.

Marinate the sweet and sour Chinese cabbage salad with it and chill for 15 minutes before serving.

TURBOT WITH SEAWEED AND ORANGE SALAD

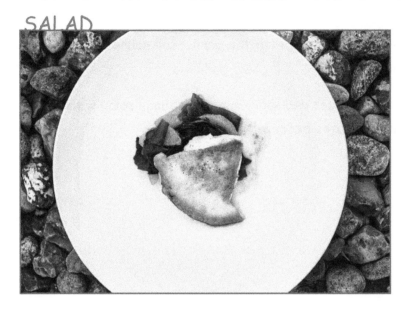

Serevings:4

INGREDIENTS

- 1.5 carton   Turbot
- 50 G   Seaweed, dried, e.g. wakame, sea spaghetti
- 2 Pc Oranges
- 2 Tbsp   sesame oil
- 2 TL Wine vinegar
- 2 TL Honey, liquid
- 2 Msp salt
- 20   ml Rapeseed oil
- 1 TL   sea-salt
- 0.5 TL   Pepper, dark, freshly ground

PREPARATION

Fillet the whole turbot. Leave the skin on the two fillets on the light side and remove the skin on the two fillets on the dark and grainy side.

Then soak the algae in cold water for 30 minutes, place in a sieve, rinse well with cold water and bring to the boil in a saucepan with plenty of water. Simmer gently for 20 minutes, then drain and let cool. Roughly cut the seaweed and place in a bowl.

Now remove the peel from the oranges with a sharp knife, remove the fillets and set aside. Squeeze the juice out of the orange meat and add to the algae. Also add sesame oil, vinegar and honey to the algae and mix well. Before serving, mix in the orange fillets and season with the 2 pinches of salt.

Cut the turbot fillets into portions. Put the rapeseed oil in a coated pan and place the fillets (those with the skin on the skin side) inside. Do not season the fillets beforehand. Now heat the pan slowly but steadily and let the fillets lie on their side until they are nice and brown and crispy (3-4 minutes).

Then turn the fillets over and reduce the temperature of the pan. Continue to cook the fillets at the remaining temperature of the pan until they are done and still have a juicy core. Season the fillets with sea salt and pepper before serving.

To serve, arrange some of the algae-orange salad in the middle of the plate and add a freshly roasted piece of fillet.

MUSTARD CRUST STEAK

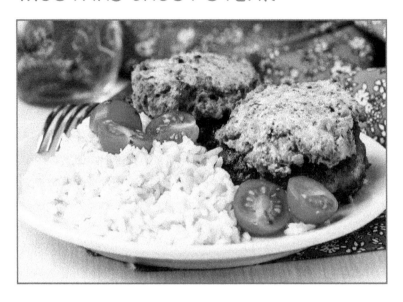

S

Serevings:4

INGREDIENTS

- 2 Tbsp   breadcrumbs
- 1 Pc egg
- 1 Tbsp   Nuts, ground
- 4 Pc Beef steaks (approx. 200 grams each)
- 8 Pc Peppercorns
- 0.5 TL   salt
- 4 Tbsp   mustard
- 4 Tbspoil

PREPARATION

Wash steaks in cold water and pat dry. Rub with freshly ground pepper. Preheat the oven to 200 degrees.

Sear the steaks in clarified butter. Let sit for 2 minutes on each side (turn only once).

Beat the egg with salt and pepper over a hot water bath until frothy. Mix in the breadcrumbs, nuts and mustard. Place the steaks in a greased casserole dish, spread the mustard mixture on the steaks, place in the oven and bake for 5 minutes.

POINTED PEPPERS FILLED WITH TOFU

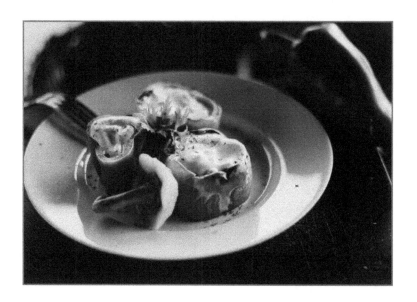

Serevings:4

INGREDIENTS

- 8 Pc Pointed peppers
- 200 ml   Vegetable broth, for the baking dish
- 1 shot Olive oil to drizzle with

for the filling

- 4 Pc spring onions
- 2 Pc   clove of garlic
- 10 Pc Cherry tomatoes
- 1 Tbsp   Olive oil, for the pan
- 160 G tofu
- 200 G Chickpeas, canned

- 1 TL   Curry powder
- 0.5 TL   Ground cumin
- 3 Tbsp   Lemon juice
- 1 Tbsp   Mint leaves, cut into strips
- 1 TL   salt
- 0.5 TL   Cayenne pepper
- 120 G Natural yoghurt

PREPARATION

Cut a lid off the top of the peppers and remove the seeds without damaging the skin.

Then clean and finely chop the spring onions. Cut the cherry tomatoes into very small pieces.

Now peel the garlic, chop it finely and sweat it together with the spring onions in a pan in hot oil for 2 minutes. Then add the tomato pieces and fry them briefly.

Cut the tofu into small pieces and add to the pan with the chickpeas, bring to the boil briefly and season with curry, caraway seeds, lemon juice, mint, salt and cayenne pepper.

Then stir in the yoghurt and pour the mixture into the peppers (with a piping nozzle) - put the pepper lid back on.

Finally, pour the vegetable stock into a baking dish, put in the filled peppers, drizzle a little olive oil and cook in a preheated oven at 180 degrees (top-bottom heat) for around 30 minutes.

POINTED PEPPERS WITH COUSCOUS

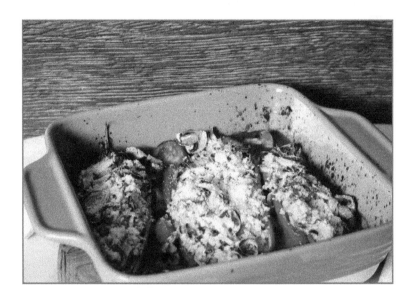

Serevings:4

INGREDIENTS

- 3 Pc leek
- 120 G couscous
- 180 ml   Vegetable broth
- 1 Pc   lemon
- 0.5 Can   Chickpeas, about 150g
- 2 Tbsp   olive oil
- 120 G Cherry tomatoes
- 180 G Mushrooms, small
- 4   Pc Pointed peppers
- 20   G Parmesan, freshly grated

for the tomato sauce

- 1 prize   salt
- 1 prize   pepper
- 2 Pc   clove of garlic
- 1 Can Tomato pieces, about 400g
- 2 TL   Oregano, dried
- 1 TL   sugar
- 2 Tbsp   Olive oil, for the pot
- 1 prize   Chilli powder

PREPARATION

First, preheat the oven to 200 ° C fan oven.

Then bring the vegetable stock to the boil in a saucepan, remove from the heat, add the couscous and let it soak for about 10 minutes - until the couscous has absorbed the stock.

In the meantime, clean and wash the leek and cut into rings. Wash the lemon with hot water, rub dry, grate the peel finely and squeeze the juice out of the lemon.

Drain the chickpeas through a sieve, rinse with cold water and drain well.

Now add half of the spring onions, chickpeas, lemon juice, lemon zest and olive oil to the couscous and mix - season with salt and pepper.

For the tomato sauce, peel the garlic, cut it into fine slices, heat it with a little oil in a small saucepan and roast it until golden brown.

Then add the tomato pieces (including juice) from the can, bring to the boil and season with oregano, chili powder, sugar and salt and pepper.

Now wash the cherry tomatoes and cut them in half. Clean and clean the mushrooms and also cut them in half. Wash the pointed peppers, pat dry, halve each lengthwise and remove the seeds.

Then put the tomato sauce in an ovenproof baking dish, spread the halved cherry tomatoes and mushrooms in it.

Fill the pepper halves with the couscous mixture and also place in the baking dish - with the filling facing up.

Finally, grate the parmesan cheese finely and sprinkle the stuffed peppers with it. Put the baking dish in the oven and bake for about 30 minutes.

POINTED CABBAGE WITH DRESSING

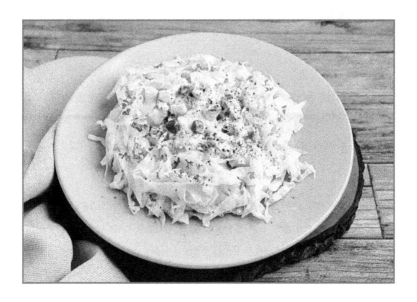

Serevings:4

INGREDIENTS

- 1200 G   cabbage
- 2000ml   Vegetable broth
- 2 Federation radish
- 2 TbspCapers
- 0.5 Federation   parsley
- 1 Pc   Medium onion
- 350 G Whole milk yogurt, creamy
- 4 Tbspmilk
- 2 prize   salt
- 2 prize   pepper
- 1 prize   sugar

PREPARATION

First remove the outer, wilted leaves from the pointed cabbage, then wash and quarter the pointed cabbage, remove the stalk and cut into strips.

Then the vegetable broth to boil in a pot and pieces of coal is in 4 portions for about 5 minutes blanch . Then remove with a slotted spoon, place in a sieve, rinse with cold water, cool and drain.

Now clean, wash and cut the radishes into small cubes. Halve the capers. Wash the parsley, shake dry, pluck the leaves from the stems and cut into strips. Peel the onion and cut into fine cubes.

Now mix the yoghurt and milk well in a bowl, stir in the radishes, capers, parsley and onions and season well with salt, pepper and sugar.

Finally, place the pointed cabbage on 4 plates, arrange the dressing in the middle and serve sprinkled with a little pepper.

ASPARAGUS WITH SALMON FILLET FROM THE STEAMER

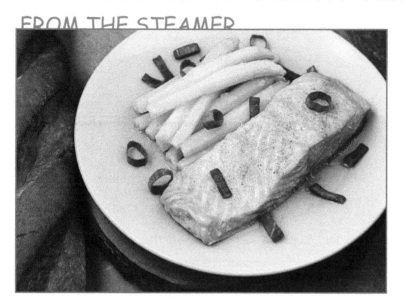

Serevings:4

INGREDIENTS

- 500 G   salmon
- 500 G Asparagus, white
- 1 prize   pepper
- 1 prize   salt
- 1 prize   sugar
- 1 Tbsp   Lemon juice
- 1 prize   Cress, finely chopped, for garnish
- 1 Pc   Spring onion

PREPARATION

First wash the white asparagus, cut off the lower woody ends, peel the asparagus and place in a perforated steamer - sprinkle with a little sugar, salt and pepper. If possible, you should choose asparagus stalks of roughly the same thickness so that they cook evenly.

Then wash the salmon fillet, pat dry, drizzle with a little lemon juice and sprinkle with salt and pepper.

Put the salmon and the finely chopped spring onions in another perforated steamer.

Now place the two steamer containers in the steamer and cook at around 90 degrees for around 15 minutes.

If the asparagus stalks are not soft after the cooking time, remove the fish and let the asparagus cook for a few more minutes.

ASPARAGUS FROM THE ROMAN POT

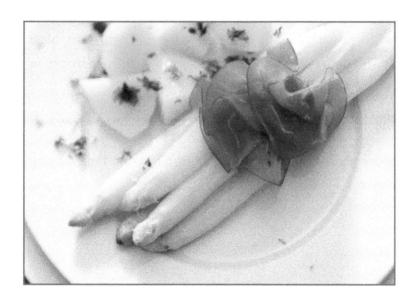

Serevings:2

INGREDIENTS

- 500 G Asparagus, white
- 1 prize   salt
- 1 prize   sugar
- 3 Tbsp   Lemon juice
- 2 Tbspwater

PREPARATION

At the beginning, water the Römertopf, ie put it in water for at least 10 minutes, this will fill the clay pores and steam will be produced during cooking.

Wash the asparagus, cut off the hard ends and peel. Season with salt, sugar and lemon juice and place in the Römertopf.

Then pour in the water and place covered in the cold oven. Now heat up to 190 degrees circulating air and cook the asparagus in the Roman pot for 60 minutes.

Tips on the recipe

If the asparagus spears are very thick, the cooking time may be a little longer.

ASPARAGUS FROM THE STEAMER WITH WILD GARLIC PESTO

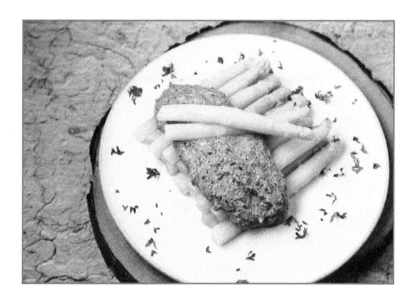

Serevings:4

INGREDIENTS

- 1 kg Asparagus, white
- 1 TL sugar

for the wild garlic pesto

- 30 G Pine nuts
- 80 G Wild garlic leaves
- 1 Federation Parsley, roughly chopped
- 30 G Parmesan cheese, grated

- 100 ml   Extra virgin olive oil
- 1 TL   Lemon juice
- 1 prize   salt
- 1 prize   pepper
- 1 Pc   Clove of garlic, peeled

PREPARATION

Peel the asparagus with an asparagus knife and cut off the woody ends (approx. 2-3 cm).

Boil the asparagus peels and the end pieces in a saucepan with water for 5 minutes.

Then layer the asparagus in the perforated steamer insert, add a little sugar and steam for about 10 minutes at 100 ° C. To do this, the steamer is filled with the asparagus water.

For the wild garlic pesto, first roast the pine nuts in a non-stick pan (without fat).

Then mix or puree the washed and chopped wild garlic, peeled garlic clove and parsley with the parmesan, pine nuts and oil.

Finally add a little lemon juice, salt and pepper and spread the pesto over the warm asparagus.

SIMPLE RAW SALAD DRESSING

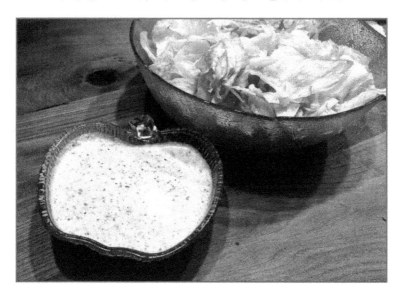

S

Serevings:1

INGREDIENTS

- 100 ml   water
- 3 Tbsp   Sunflower seeds
- 0.5 Pc lemon
- 1 Pc   clove of garlic
- 2 Tbsp   6 herb mixture
- 1 prize   salt and pepper

PREPARATION

First, squeeze the lemon half, peel the garlic and chop it roughly.

Then put lemon juice, garlic, water, sunflower seeds, herbs and salt and pepper in a small blender and puree for 30 seconds.

SELLERY SOUP

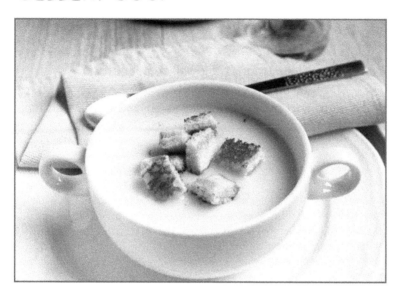

S

Servings:4

INGREDIENTS

- Pc onion
- 500 G   celery root
- 25 G butter
- 700 ml   Vegetable broth
- 200 ml   Milk, low fat
- 1 prize   salt
- 1 prize pepper
- 1 Msp nutmeg

PREPARATION

Wash, peel and cut the celery into large pieces. Peel the onions, chop them finely and sauté them in a saucepan with butter.

Then add the broth, celery, salt, pepper and nutmeg and cook covered for about 20 minutes at a lower temperature.

Then add the milk and puree the soup with the hand blender. Season again to taste and just warm up more.

CONCLUSION

If you want to lose a few pounds, the low-carb and low-fat diet will eventually reach your limits. Although the weight can be reduced with the diets, the success is usually only short-lived because the diets are too one-sided. So if you want to lose weight and avoid a classic yo-yo effect, you should rather check your energy balance and recalculate your daily calorie requirement.

The ideal is to adhere to a gentle variant of the low-fat diet with 60 to 80 grams of fat per day for life. It helps to maintain the weight and protects against diabetes and high blood lipids with all their health risks.

The low-fat diet is comparably easy to implement because you only have to forego fatty foods or severely limit their proportion of the daily amount of food. With the low-carb diet, on the other hand, much more precise planning and more stamina are necessary. Anything that really fills you up is usually high in carbohydrates and should be avoided. Under certain circumstances, this can lead to food cravings and thus to failure of the diet. It is essential that you eat properly. Many statutory health insurance companies therefore offer prevention courses or pay you for individual nutritional advice. Such advice is extremely important, especially if you decide on a weight-loss diet in which you want to permanently change your entire diet. Whether your private health insurance pays for such measures depends on the tariff you have taken out. In the meantime, however, individual nutritional advice has been taken over by many private providers.

DETOX DIET

INTRODUCTION

Cleaning the body appears to be a major preventive measure to health problems. Because most of us are busy, and unable or unwilling to maintain a strict diet, we have to do it all ourselves. The body has built up chemical's day after day. We do not notice side effects because the chemicals are harmless in small amounts, but dangerous in larger amounts. A proper and balanced diet is necessary to relieve toxins and chemicals and maintain a healthy and normal life.

A detox diet's main idea is to limit consumption of most foods and only drink water and vegetables for a few days. Most programmes then allow for slow re-introduction of other foods. The diets generally restrict foods that are said to have harmful toxins. Besides, a detox diet should also remove toxins from the body. The detox diet helps the liver and other organs clean up the toxins. We produce sweat, faeces, and urine.

Our bodies cannot cope with the normal daily consumption of chemicals. The chemicals come from food, as well as a wide variety of other sources. It is unclear what is causing the disease, but it is believed that pesticides, heavy metals, such as mercury and lead, and the chemicals in cigarettes and the air we breathe all cause an excess build up. The smaller amounts of these chemicals are harmless. The excessive intake and build up can lead to disease.

A popular detox diet is the combination of nothing but fruits and water. Supplements, herbs and vitamins can be used to metabolise certain chemicals in our bodies. Some supplements will help mobilise toxins in fat and other toxin deposits throughout the body. Sauna therapies help the body rid itself of chemicals through sweat. There are many other diets and detox programmes that are also effective. Regular body detoxification is a preventative action that promotes a healthier future.

A plan for a detox diet is not aimed at weight loss. Combining natural organic food, herbs, and simple exercises to purge the body of accumulated toxins aims to cleanse and revitalise the body. Consumption of processed foods, non-vegetarian foods, and sugars over time leads to the clogging of waste matter from the colon's inner walls. This causes internal cleansing organs such as the liver and kidneys to be overloaded. They become sluggish, allowing the toxins and bacteria to re-enter the circulatory system through faeces, urine or sweat instead of total elimination. These toxins can lead to fatigue, skin and other organ infections, migraines, flatulence, heartburn, constipation and many other serious illnesses. A regular detox diet plan can remove the accumulated toxins from the body and lead to an active life free of illness.

This diet is not intended for people with diabetes, patients with low blood pressure, anorexic individuals or adolescents, as it does not provide sufficient fuel for their physical activity. It can be a weeklong diet of liquids, organic raw fruits and vegetables to cleanse the system. Reintroducing other foods gradually, but refraining from consuming non-vegetarian and processed foods. It is possible to use certain natural herbs, too.

CHAPTER ONE
What is detoxification

Detoxification is the natural process of eliminating and neutralizing toxins from the body. The colon, lungs, liver, kidneys, skin are the organs that play an important role in detoxification.

What does detoxification mean?

Detoxification has been known since ancient Egypt. Doctors then talked about detoxification, showing patients that diseases accompanied by pain, fatigue cannot be treated without a detoxification treatment.

Today it has been shown that even the best treatment methods do not give lasting results without a detoxification treatment. You can successfully treat with a detoxification cure intestinal transit disorders, constipation, bloating , allergies, chronic fatigue, tired liver! You can lose 2-3 extra pounds with a detox cure! You can forget about headaches, joint pain with the help of a detox cure!

At the same time, today, the detoxification cure is a new trend in beauty. Hollywood stars - Cindy Crawford, Oprah, Gwen Stefani, Liv Tyler - have made detoxification a way of life. They use detoxification belts and, in particular, colon cleansing belts as a method of disease prevention and as a method of beautification, of losing extra pounds.

Detoxification mechanisms

Normally, our body has a natural ability to detoxify. The main mechanisms of detoxification of the body are the colon, lungs, liver, kidneys, skin.

These organs fulfil the detoxification mission, eliminating toxins from foods contaminated with pesticides, herbicides, chemical fertilizers, hormones, antibiotics, E-foods, polluted air.

Unfortunately, in many cases, the body's detoxification capacity is exceeded. The colon, liver, kidneys, lungs, and skin are no longer able to effectively eliminate toxins due to unbalanced diet, stress and pollution, so detoxification is necessary.

Toxins accumulate in the body. Suppose we do not follow a detoxification treatment. In that case, there are first bloating, flatulence, poor digestion, slow intestinal transit, constipation, weight gain, allergies, concentration disorders, headaches, depression, and unpleasant odour body, breath.

Why is detoxification of the body important?

We hear more and more often about our detoxification, ideas, concepts, cures and diets. Detoxification is an alternative treatment that aims to eliminate toxins and substances accumulated in the body that can negatively affect the short or long term. Both nutritionists and doctors recommend it. However, before starting a detox program it is important to know "WHY?" Detoxify our body before we know what a detox involves and how to do it.

The human body functions as a machine that, uncleaned from time to time, collects toxic substances that lead to health problems. Every day, our body comes in contact with toxins that we find in different forms: cleaning products, alcoholic beverages, cigarette smoke, pollution, in make-up products, perfumes, etc. Also, some toxic substances are not as "visible", being found in the form of pesticides and herbicides on fruits and vegetables that are not washed before consumption and, at the same time, in the form of additives prepackaged products.

All this affects the proper functioning of the organs in the human body. Unlike other parts of our body, it is very difficult to know how well the liver works, and this is exactly the main detoxifying organ. In addition to the synthesis and secretion of bile, the liver acts as a filter for toxins and bacteria in the blood. It chemically neutralizes toxins, turning them into substances that the kidneys can eliminate.

Most of the molecules produced by our body every day are to get rid of waste products. We need hundreds of enzymes, vitamins and other molecules to help the body get rid of unwanted waste and chemicals. Although most of the work is done by the liver and intestinal tract, the kidneys, lungs, lymphatic system and skin are involved in this complex detoxification system.

We can help the body through various cures and diets with fruits, vegetables, teas or food supplements. However, doctors warn that detoxification is not for everyone and advise people suffering from kidney disease, diabetes, anemia to be careful when opting for such a treatment.

Nutradose Detox is a dietary supplement made from natural extracts of dandelion, apples, artichokes, red cabbage, parsley, grapefruit seeds and buckwheat. These ingredients make up a unique cocktail, 100% natural, which gives the body a state of well-being, purification ensuring a state of health by reducing water retention and eliminating toxins.

Among the natural extracts listed above, we mention parsley as known for its role in purifying and cleansing the body of toxins, being a powerful antioxidant; Red cabbage has antioxidant properties through its rich content of flavonoids and phyto-antioxidants that stimulate the production of essential enzymes to maintain normal metabolic functions in the body. Grapefruit also contains bioflanoids that prevent the deposition of cholesterol and help improve digestion, intensifying the liver's activity and normalizing substances in the body.

Do Detox Diets Work?

Some people report feeling more concentrated and energetic during and after detox diets. However, this may be partly because a detox diet eliminates highly processed foods with solid fats and added sugars. Avoiding these nutrient-rich foods with low nutrition for a few days may be part of the reason why people feel better.

On the other hand, many people also report feeling very bad during the detox period.

The main health risks of detox diets relate to severe energy restrictions and nutritional inadequacy.

CHAPTER TWO
What Are Toxins

In recent years, all the media (including magazines, the news, and even movies and television shows) have been focused on toxins, detox diets, or the best way to exercise. However, most people still do not know what toxins are or why it is a good idea to purify our body.

Things like toxins are called harmful substances because they get inside cells, whether plants, animals, or bacteria. For some people, the symptoms do not appear right away. The symptoms may slowly develop over time.

In terms of toxins, you may be concerned that there is damage when the toxins are allowed to accumulate in the body. We explore where these toxins come from, and what we can do to prevent their entering our air or water.

What are toxins?

As we have mentioned, toxins are substances that are potentially harmful to our cells and tissues. They can be small molecules, proteins or other elements from both outside and inside the body.

First of all, we must know that toxins are generated in our body all the time, due to the metabolic processes that we need to survive. For example, the mechanism by which our cells obtain energy generates free radicals.

Free radicals are unstable molecules that are considered toxins, since they can cause damage cells if they accumulate. We also generate numerous toxins when we eat, breathe or consume a substance such as tobacco.

What happens is that we have mechanisms that allow us to neutralize all these toxins or eliminate them. When they are neutralized, they are prevented from reaching very high levels, which is harmful to tissues.

The two most important organs in the neutralization and elimination of toxins are the liver and the kidney. Through urine and feces we expel a large part of them.

It is essential that these organs work as they should, so that the purification is correct. Kidney and liver diseases alter the detoxification process and delay the elimination of free radicals, affecting aging, for example.

How to recognize when the body needs cleansing? Symptoms

- Lack of energy
- Slow metabolism
- Inability to shed unnecessary kilograms
- Skin problems
- Matte and brittle hair and nails
- Intestinal problems and digestive disorders
- Problems with concentration and memory
- Headaches
- Bad breath
- Wrapped tongue
- Heartburn
- Problems with menstruation

- Insomnia
- A tendency to worry about everything and mood swings
- Cellulitis
- Depression
- No creativity
- Reluctance to change

The above symptoms indicate that our body is overloaded and needs help in getting rid of harmful substances. However, we often drown out a call for help.

This is because we have become a habit of sipping another coffee instead of taking a break to rest, drinking soda to recharge our batteries, and raising our energy levels with unhealthy sugar.

We can easily stay at work after hours, and we do not have the strength to find a few minutes for gymnastics. Rather spend time standing in line to see the doctor, and then spend your money on medication, rather than rest for an hour on a meditation cushion and stock up on healthy food. Cleansing the body should be a priority for all of us.

The Most Common Ways to Detox

If you know your body and the risks you are taking by using material-related products, you can be more certain to keep your body free of toxins and improve health.

We will tell you what foods you should eat and ways you can exercise daily to improve your life quality.

It should not be detoxifying the body by taking it in one day intensively. Or by using a cleansing product. It should continue to be active in the system for a longer period, not taken in very large amounts. It will also not have any effect if the person stops taking it or stops taking it when he/she stops.

On a day to day basis it is a mix of knowing what to avoid, and what types of treatments can help us. An easy way to change your lifestyle is to start eating healthier.

- **Increase the daily intake of fruits and vegetables**

Try to eat at least 3 or more vegetables and 2 or more servings of fresh fruit every day, although ideally you should have 8-10 servings of fruit and vegetables each day.

- **Use natural sweeteners**

Eliminate sugar from your diet. You can get the sweet taste with all-natural sugar substitutes like stevia or honey.

- **Try foods rich in probiotics**

Probiotic foods are rich in live microorganisms that help improve digestion, the functioning of the immune system, and decrease inflammation.

The most common probiotics are: Lactobacillus acidophilus in the small intestine and Bifidobacterium bifidum in the large intestine.

We can find them in products like kefir and yogurt, and they are also available in supplement form.

- **Whole grains**

Brown rice, quinoa, oats, millet, amaranth or buckwheat are some examples of foods that will help you improve your intestine's functioning and, therefore, help you eliminate excess toxins.

- **Drink more fluids**

Most of us don't drink enough. Water is essential for optimal digestive function, and it is especially important to drink enough fluids, especially if we are going to increase fibre intake. Drinking fluids plays a very important role in daily detoxification. Liquids help flush toxins through the organs more efficiently.

Try to drink 8-10 glasses of water each day. We can increase the amount of liquid we drink daily with infusions, broths, ...

- **Foods rich in fiber**

If you are not getting enough fiber, you will not help your body eliminate leftover products as you should through digestion.

Fiber is a very important part of a healthy diet and can be found in fruits, vegetables, and legumes.

- **Foods rich in omega-3 fatty acids**

In fish such as anchovies, herring, mackerel, sardines and salmon, in avocado and flax seed it will make the digestive process smoother, helping purify the body.

- **Substitute green tea for coffee**

A cup of coffee doesn't have to be harmful. The problem arises when we drink too much coffee every day. We do not know the effect that excess caffeine can have on our body in the long term.

The green tea is rich in antioxidants that can help eliminate toxins from the body and contain caffeine, which Is negligible.

- **Eliminate bad habits**

Like smoking or drinking alcohol.

- **Practice physical exercise**

Exercise is one of the best ways to detoxify the body.

- **make sleeping a priority**

Getting a good night's sleep can also help eliminate toxin build-up, especially since your organs are "recharged" and ready to do their job.

Essential foods to cleanse the body

- **Apples.**

They are excellent at detoxifying the body, and apple juice helps to cope with viruses' effects when we catch an infection, such as the flu. Apples contain pectin, which helps to effectively remove heavy metal compounds and other toxins from the body. It is no coincidence that pectin is included in detoxification programs to treat drug addicts using heroin, cocaine, marijuana. Also, apples help eliminate intestinal parasites, certain skin diseases, help treat inflammation of the bladder, and prevent liver problems.

- **Beets.**

The main "cleaner" of our body from toxins and other "unnecessary" substances is the liver. And beets naturally help detoxify the liver itself. Beets, like apples, contain a lot of pectin. Many doctors recommend that you constantly eat beets in all forms - boiled, baked, stewed, use them in the preparation of savoury dishes and desserts.

- **Celery.**

Indispensable for detoxification. It helps cleanse the blood, prevents uric acid deposition in the joints, and stimulates the thyroid and pituitary glands. Celery also acts as a mild diuretic, making it easier for the kidneys and bladder to function.

- **Onion.**

Promotes the elimination of toxins through the skin. Also, it cleanses the intestines.

- **Cabbage.**

Its anti-inflammatory properties have been known for a long time. Cabbage juice is used as a remedy for stomach ulcers. And lactic acid. Which cabbage contains helps to keep the colon healthy. Like other cruciferous vegetables, cabbage contains sulphorphane, a substance that helps the body fight toxins.

- **Garlic.**

Contains allicin, which helps eliminate toxins and contributes to the maintenance of normal white blood cells. Garlic cleanses the respiratory system and purifies the blood. Lesser-known property: It helps eliminate nicotine from the body and can be a great addition to your diet when you quit smoking.

- **Artichoke.**

Just like beets, it is good for the liver, as it stimulates bile secretion. Plus, artichokes are high in antioxidants and fiber.

- **Lemon.**

It is recommended to drink lemon juice, adding it to warm water, such lemonade is a tonic for the liver and heart. Also, it prevents the formation of alkaline kidney stones. A large amount of vitamin C helps to cleanse the vascular system.

- **Ginger.**

Its anti-cold properties are widely known. But the diaphoretic effect of ginger simultaneously allows the body to expel toxins through the skin.

- **Carrots.**

Carrots and carrot juice help in the treatment of respiratory, skin diseases. They are used to treat anemia and to regulate the menstrual cycle.

- **Water.**

All our tissues and cells need water to function well. Even our mental health depends on the amount of water we drink. When the body is dehydrated, it negatively affects all bodily functions.

Modern man has lost the habit of drinking pure water, replacing it with coffee, tea, and sweet soda. As a result, in the United States, about 75% of the population is chronically dehydrated. Thus, increasing water consumption (modern nutritionists consider 1.5 - 2 liters per day to be the norm) is an important task.

How effective are detox diets?

Detox diets are more popular nowadays than ever. There are whole programs, trainings and detox nutrition schemes. Detox becomes especially relevant after the holidays. But is it good to kick start detoxification? Let's analyse in this material.

Detox diets differ in the types of foods that need to be limited and in duration. A typical detox diet consists of a fasting period and a strict diet (fruits, vegetables, fruit juices, water). Sometimes complete starvation is introduced, herbal infusions, teas are used, and enemas are sometimes added.

It is believed that detox diets remove harmful substances from the body, improve energy distribution in the body, improve concentration and mood. The positive effects are probably associated with a change in diet (fast carbohydrates, trans fats are excluded, the concentration of vitamins increases). However, there are no specific studies that would prove this claim.

The excretory system functions in the body - the liver, kidneys, skin. Accordingly, the body can get rid of "toxins" through urine, feces and sweat. Substances that are not easily eliminated from the body include persistent organic pollutants (POPs), phthalates, bisphenol

A (BPA) and heavy metals. They accumulate in adipose tissue or blood and take a long time to get rid of. However, at present, they are less and less often found in food. This means that in this case, detox is not effective.

There is an opinion that detox will help you lose weight, but this topic is not well understood. With detox diets, the body most likely loses its supply of carbohydrates and fluids, not fat. After the end of the detox, the pounds often return.

If you want to follow a detox diet, you should first consult with your doctor and consider the side effects. Detox diets that severely limit protein intake are detrimental to the body. Prolonged fasting leads to fatigue and vitamin and mineral deficiencies. Bowel cleansing can cause cramping, bloating, nausea, and vomiting.

You should always eat a healthy diet for lasting results - vegetables and fruits, whole grains, and lean protein sources.

Benefits of a Diet to Detoxify the Body

- **Increase your Energy**

Many followers of detox programs report that they feel more energetic. This makes sense because as you detox, you stop eating things that made you need a detox in the first place. By cutting out sugar, caffeine, trans fat, saturated fat and replacing them with fresh fruits and vegetables, you will have a natural energy charge, one that comes without the power outage afterwards. It is important to stay well hydrated while on a detox program, and this can also be a source of increased energy if you don't usually drink a lot of water during the day.

- **Rid the Body of Excess Waste**

The biggest thing with which a diet can detoxify the body helps to allow the body to get rid of any excess waste it is accumulating. Most detox programs are designed to encourage the body to cleanse itself, detoxifying the liver, kidneys and colon to work better. Cleaning the colon is an important part of the detoxification process because these toxins need to leave the body. A colon full of toxins can reintroduce them into the body instead of eliminating them. Eating fruits and vegetables even after detox is a good way to keep things going.

- **Help with Weight Loss**

It's easy to see how a detox can make you lose weight in the short term, but a healthier way to look at it would be to establish long-term eating habits and get rid of unhealthy habits. It is often the drastic reduction in calories and rapid weight loss that gains focus, especially in the media. Short-term results won't last if you don't trade bad food for good, and use your energy to exercise more and be more active.

- **Stronger Immune System**

When you go on a diet to detoxify the body, you free your organs to work as they should. This helps to improve your immune system as you will be able to absorb nutrients better, including Vitamin C. Many of the herbs you take in the detox will help the lymphatic system, which plays a big role in maintaining your health. Many detox programs focus on light exercise to help circulate lymph fluid through the body and help to strengthen your immune system in the process.

- **Better skin**

Your skin is your biggest organ, so it makes sense that it shows positive results with a detox program. One way to help your detox efforts is to take a sauna to help your body eliminate more toxins through sweat. You can expect cleaner, smoother skin at the end of your detox plan. It has also been reported that detoxification can help with acne, although the condition may worsen before it gets better as toxins are released. You may feel your skin itch before it gets clean, but this is part of the process and a sign that you are on the right track.

- **Better breath**

When detoxing with colon cleanses, follow a programme that includes a colon cleanse so that the toxins may be flushed out of the body. Experts have a theory that bad breath may come from a colon full of toxins or bacteria. Once you can clean your digestive system, you may be able to return to some sort of proper eating habits, and your breath may improve. You should be aware that your breath may worsen during the detox, but when it ends, it will turn around positively. This will occur naturally. It is a normal part of the manufacturing of the product.

- **Promotes Health Changes**

It is difficult to change an old habit, and a detox program - no matter how long - is a way to put a barrier between your old habits and your new ones. If you are addicted to sugar, caffeine, fried foods, you can use a detox program to help you eliminate those cravings. Often, if you just try to stop eating these foods or drinks, you will have limited success and return to old habits. But if you cleanse your body and exchange these foods for healthier choices, you may be more likely to continue with your new habits.

- **Clearer Thinking**

A good detox diet will pay attention to your mental state while cleaning. The use of meditation is often recommended to reconnect to your body during this cleansing time. Detox followers often say that they lose the feeling of mental fog and think more clearly during a detox. It makes sense, since many sugary or fatty foods that surround us daily make us feel lethargic and influence our thoughts' quality.

- **Healthier Hair**

When you can see your hair, it is already considered dead, since its growth occurs in the hair follicle. That is why it is important to keep your body running at full steam during a detox program. When your hair can grow without being inhibited by internal toxins, you will see and feel the difference. In many cases, hair is shinier and softer to the touch. Detoxifying is not enough to prevent hair loss, but many people report that their hair grows faster, a sign of healthier hair.

- **Feeling of Lightness**

One of the possible benefits of being a person who is on a detoxification programme is a feeling of lightness. There are many reasons that this might be happening, especially if the person is doing a colon cleanse as part of the programme When you eat in an environment that supports a balanced diet and replace old foods with the freshest, most organic, healthiest foods; you will feel a lot lighter Also it is extremely important not to overeat in the detox as it can make you feel light as well, and it will give you the energy you miss.

- **Anti-Age Benefits**

The constant amount of toxins the body has to deal with is one of the aging process's contributing factors. By reducing the amount of free radical damage to your body, you will have short-term benefits and long-term benefits and more longevity. When you finish your detox program, it is very important not to go back to the lifestyle that was causing the toxins. Staying on a better diet and doing activities daily are great ways to make sure you always feel good.

- **Better feeling of well-being**

When you do a detox, you feel good, and when you feel good, good things happen. Detoxifying is often used strategically to lose weight or start a diet, but there is no better reason than just to feel better. When you set the stage for feeling good, you will improve all areas of your life, and you should see better relationships, more productivity at work and a new joy in living.

Who shouldn't detoxify the body?

It is worth remembering that detoxification is not recommended for everyone, If one of the following situations occurs, before starting the cleansing process, consult a doctor:

- You are a child
- You are pregnant or breastfeeding
- Recently, psychiatric or psychotherapeutic treatment has been completed
- Drugs are taken
- You are recovering from a serious illness

Side effects of detoxification of the body

Importantly, the body cleansing program is intended to bring maximum health benefits with a minimum of side effects. These reactions are completely normal, they occur in most people and pass quickly, and they certainly indicate that the body is getting rid of toxins. The side effects include:

- Fatigue
- Constipation
- Intestinal relaxation
- Frequent bowel movements and increased stool indifference
- Headaches
- Wrapped tongue
- Increased sweating
- Skin spots and blemishes
- Changes in urination
- Runny nose and runny nose

- Anger and irritability

What foods to eat and avoid

What to consume	What not to consume
Fresh fruit	Fried food
Vegetables	Processed foods (white flour)
Vegetables	Sugar
Rice	Excess common salt
Quinoa	Caffeine
Oats	Soft drinks
Natural teas	Alcoholic beverages
Legumes	Food with dyes
Chestnuts	Milks and derivatives
Sea salt	Sweetener
Cocoa powder	High fructose corn syrup
Free-range eggs	Saturated fat and trans fat

CHAPTER THREE
Detox Diet Meal Plan

3-day detox diet: example menu

First day:

- Breakfast: fruit salad and dried fruit
- Lunch: brown rice and cooked vegetables
- Dinner: fresh vegetable salad

Second day:

- Breakfast: whole grain oatmeal, fresh fruit
- Lunch: salad of raw vegetables and legumes
- Snack: fresh fruit salad
- Dinner: brown rice and cooked potatoes

Third day:

- Breakfast: centrifuged fruit and vegetables
- Lunch: quinoa and legumes
- Snack: fresh fruit salad
- Dinner: vegetable and dried fruit salad

7-day detox diet: sample menu

Monday

- Breakfast: low-fat yogurt and a banana
- Lunch: vegetable and tuna salad
- Snack: 100 grams of berries
- Dinner: steamed fish with vegetables

Tuesday

- Breakfast: a cup of almond milk and a fruit
- Lunch: 50g of brown rice and legumes
- Dinner: 100g of defatted chicken breast and vegetable salad

Wednesday

- Breakfast: a fruit salad, Greek yogurt and 30 grams of dried fruit
- Lunch: 100 grams of steamed fish and 50 grams of quinoa
- Dinner: mixed salad and potatoes

Thursday

- Breakfast: rolled oats and a handful of nuts
- Lunch: 100 grams of defatted turkey and steamed vegetables
- Dinner: 80g of wholemeal pasta with tomato sauce and fresh basil.

Friday

- Breakfast: a glass of fruit salad
- Lunch: 80 grams of wholemeal pasta and tomato sauce
- Snack: 30 grams of dried fruit

- Dinner: vegetable soup and 1 fruit

Saturday

- Breakfast: low-fat yogurt and a fruit
- Lunch: salad of mixed vegetables and legumes
- Snack: a glass of fruit salad
- Dinner: 100g of baked salmon and potatoes

Sunday

- Breakfast: rolled oats and a seasonal fruit
- Lunch: 100 grams of lean meat and grilled vegetables
- Dinner: 80 grams of wholemeal pasta and legumes

FAQ about detox diets

1. What is a detox diet?

In the detox diet, foods are specifically added to the body that promote the detoxification process. Everything that can make you sick permanently is avoided. This includes, for example, an unhealthy diet, but also stress or harmful environmental influences. In this way, the body should be strengthened from the inside out - and the fasting person should feel good and fit again on a holistic level after the detox diet.

2. How long does a detox cycle take?

There are detox cures from 3 or 5 days. To achieve good health results and lose a little weight, you should plan at least a week's stay. A 14-day detox vacation (or even more) is often offered and is a great opportunity to free yourself from stress on all levels, both physically and mentally.

3. Which foods are on the plate during a detox cure?

You can expect many fruit and vegetables, lots of colorful juice, vegetable broth, smoothies, soups, herbal teas and of course water. The detox diet doesn't have to be boring! Alcohol, coffee, tobacco and meat are prohibited during the fast.

4. Can I also do the detox diet at home?

We recommend taking the cure in a hotel specially designed for detoxification. The doctors will examine you initially and accompany you the entire time. Also, an individual detox diet plan will be created for you. You will be given relevant knowledge during a nutritional consultation, which you can take home with you after your health vacation and integrate it into everyday life.

5. What are the side effects of this diet?

By throwing eating habits overboard during the detox cure that may have been programmed for years, side effects such as headaches, weakness or bad mood can occur, especially in the first few days. This is precisely why it is nice to take the cure in a hotel, as you are not alone in your project. Also, the hotels offer the perfect infrastructure for fasting and offer a great supporting program. Most of our fasting hotels are also located amid fabulous natural landscapes, which quickly make the initial side effects evaporate.

6. Who shouldn't undergo a detox?

Since the detox cure is not a zero diet and the body is supplied with important minerals and plant substances, there are initially no health concerns. However, if you suffer from acute infections, cancer, severe cardiovascular diseases, mental illnesses or an eating disorder, we advise against the detox cure. In all cases, if in any doubt, you should be honest with yourself and seek advice from your doctor. Pregnant women are not allowed to fast.

CHAPTER FOUR
Recipes for Detoxification

Mango detox juice

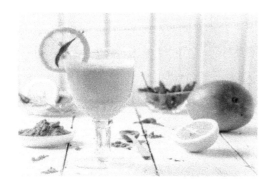

- Cooking time 5 to 15 min
- servings 4

ingredients

4-5 mangoes (ripe)

1 lemon

1 piece of ginger (the size of a thumb)

1 pod (s) chilli (red)

1 tbsp turmeric (ground)

preparation

1. For the mango detox juice, peel and core the ripe mangoes. Also remove the lemon and ginger from the peel. Remove the seeds from the chilli pepper and squeeze through a juicer along with the remaining prepared ingredients.
2. Stir turmeric into the finished mango detox juice and serve.

Thyme turkey with red wine lentils

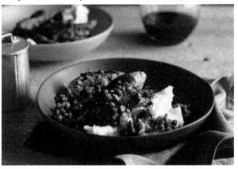

- Cooking time 30 to 60 min
- servings 4

ingredients

- 4 turkey fillets (150g each)
- 1/2 bunch of thyme
- 1 onion (red)
- 1 tbsp rapeseed oil
- 200 g lentils
- 1/8 l red wine
- salt
- pepper

preparation

1. Preheat the oven to 200 ° C. Salt and pepper the turkey fillets and wrap them in aluminum foil with thyme sprigs and cook in the oven for 20 minutes. Simultaneously, cook the lentils in unsalted water according to the package instructions (do not cook completely).

2. Peel the onion, cut into thin rings and sauté briefly in a saucepan with a little oil. Pour red wine on top, salt and pepper and then finish cooking together with the lentils (without cooking water) and fresh thyme (simply pluck from the branch).

3. Your detox foods: thyme, onion, canola, lentils, and red wine

Cabbage soup "Asia Style"

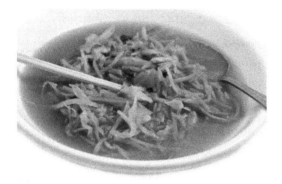

- Cooking time 30 to 60 min
- servings 4

Ingredients

- 1 head of white cabbage (small)
- 1 teaspoon paprika powder (sweet)
- 1 carrot
- 2 pcs. Onions
- 3 toe (s) of garlic
- 2 tbsp olive oil
- 1 pod (s) of chilli
- 1 stick (s) lemongrass
- 1 tuber (s) of ginger (large)
- 1 tbsp caraway seeds (ground)
- 1000 ml vegetable stock (alternatively organic soup powder and water)
- 500 ml green tea
- salt

preparation

1. For the "Asia Style" cabbage soup, first halve the cabbage, remove the stalk and cut into fine strips. Peel the carrot (in strips), onions, lemongrass and garlic and cut into small pieces. Prepare green tea. Heat the oil in a large saucepan, add the carrots, onions and garlic and sauté briefly.

2. Add white cabbage and roast briefly. Remove the pan from the heat, add the paprika powder, lemongrass, freshly grated ginger, chilli pepper and caraway seeds and stir. Pour the vegetable stock and green tea on top. Simmer on low heat for 20 minutes.

3. Before serving the "Asia Style" cabbage soup, remove the chilli pepper and season to taste again.

Goji curd cream

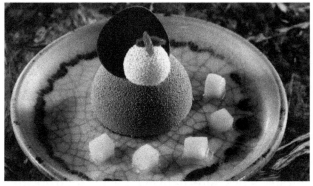

ingredients

- 250 g low-fat curd cheese (creamy)
- 100 ml soy milk
- 20 g hazelnuts (grated)

- 1 tbsp flaxseed (crushed)
- 1 teaspoon maple syrup
- 20 g goji berries (dried)

preparation

1. Beat the skimmed curd cheese with soy milk until smooth.
2. Mix in the hazelnuts, flax seeds and maple syrup.
3. Sprinkle the goji berries on top and serve the cream.

Pasta detoxicant

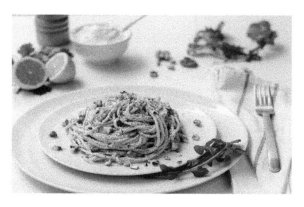

- Cooking time 30 to 60 min
- Servings 4

ingredients

- 2 jars of anchovies
- 100 g capers (medium)
- 50 g cranberries (dried, cranberries)
- 40 g pine nuts
- 2 glass artichoke hearts

- 500 g whole wheat pasta (without egg)
- 1 tbsp oregano

preparation

1. Prepare salted cooking water for the pasta. Cook the pasta al dente according to the instructions.
2. Brown the pine nuts in a non-fat non-stick pan.
3. Cut the anchovies, capers and artichoke hearts into small pieces.
4. Use the oil from a glass in which the anchovies were pickled for your sauce: mix the oil, the anchovies, the capers, the artichoke hearts, the cranberries, the pine nuts and the oregano into a mass and briefly heat the sauce.
5. Serve the pasta with the sauce.

Brown rice pudding

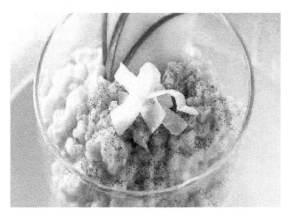

- Cooking time 30 to 60 min
- servings 4

ingredients

- 2 apples
- 100 g short grain rice (natural)
- 50 ml soy milk

- 200 ml of water
- 40 g almonds (natural)
- 30 g raisins
- 1 pinch of cinnamon (ground)
- 1 pair of cloves
- 1 tbsp honey
- 150 g low-fat curd cheese (creamy)

preparation

1. For the brown rice pudding, cook rice with 200 ml of water in a covered saucepan (about 40 minutes according to the instructions) over medium heat. In the meantime, peel, core and cut the apples into rings and cook them briefly with the cloves in a little water until the rings are soft.
2. Once the cooking time is up and the rice has absorbed the water, remove the lid and add soy milk, nuts, raisins, honey and cinnamon. Now take the pot off the stove, let the rice cool down briefly and mix the curd cheese into the mixture.
3. Now alternate layers of apple rings and rice mixture in a glass. Finish with an apple ring and dust the rice pudding with a little cinnamon.

Potato and turmeric herb

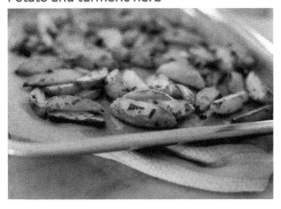

- Cooking time 30 to 60 min
- servings 4

ingredients

- 500 g sauerkraut (pre-cooked)
- 60 g apricots (dried)
- 60 g lentils (black)
- 600 g potatoes (floury)
- 250 g vegetable soup (organic, soup cubes)
- 1 teaspoon paprika powder (sweet)
- 1 teaspoon caraway seeds
- 1 teaspoon turmeric (ground, turmeric)
- 1 tbsp curry powder
- 1 onion (white)
- 1 tbsp olive oil

preparation

1. For the potato and turmeric herb, prepare the vegetable soup with 250 ml of water and half an organic vegetable soup cube.
2. Peel and dice the potatoes and onions.

3. Sauté the onion in a large saucepan with oil for 2 minutes, mix in the paprika powder and pour the vegetable stock on top.
4. Add potatoes, lentils (the cooking time of lentils may vary), caraway seeds, turmeric and curry powder and cook covered for 20 minutes on a low flame.
5. Finally add the chopped apricots and the cabbage and leave the pan on the stove for another 3 to 4 minutes.

Colourful curry chicken skewers

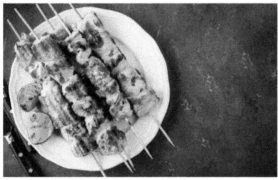

- Cooking time 15 to 30 min
- Servings 4

ingredients

- 600 g chicken fillet (skinless)
- 1 banana (large, unripe)
- 1 onion (white)
- 1 pc. Paprika (yellow)
- 1 packet of cocktail tomatoes
- 1 tbsp curry powder
- salt and pepper

- Wooden skewers

preparation

1. For the colorful curry chicken skewers, preheat the oven to 200 ° C. Cut the chicken into small cubes.
2. Peel the onion and banana and cut into small slices.
3. Cut the bell pepper into small square pieces and
4. halve the cherry tomatoes.
5. Alternate all ingredients on the skewers.
6. Salt, pepper and sprinkle generously with curry powder. Place the curry chicken skewers on a baking sheet lined with baking paper and bake in the oven at 200 ° C for about 12 minutes.

Hot strawberry buttermilk

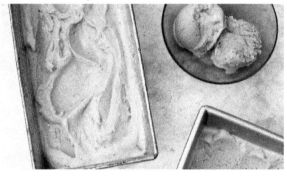

- Cooking time 15 to 30 min
- Servings 4

ingredients

- 200 ml low-fat buttermilk (natural)
- 1 teaspoon maple syrup
- 125 g strawberries (fresh or frozen)
- 1 pinch of cayenne pepper

preparation

1. For the hot strawberry buttermilk, wash the strawberries, remove the stalk, cut in half and puree with the maple syrup, cayenne pepper and a few tablespoons of water.
2. Pour the cold buttermilk into a glass and pour the puree over it.

Spaghetti vegginese

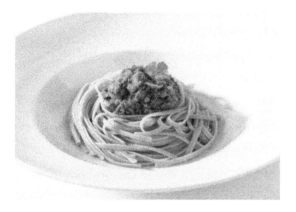

- Cooking time 30 to 60 min
- Servings 4

ingredients

- 400 g whole wheat spaghetti
- 150 g soy granules
- 200 g carrots
- 1 pc. Paprika (yellow)
- 1 kg tomatoes (strained)
- 1 onion (white)
- 50 g capers (small)
- 100 g olives (green, seedless)
- 4 pieces of garlic cloves
- 4 tbsp tomato paste

- 250 ml red wine (strong)
- 6 drops of Tabasco sauce
- 1/2 bunch of parsley
- 1 tbsp oregano
- 1 teaspoon paprika powder (sweet)
- 1/2 teaspoon cinnamon
- 1 tbsp olive oil
- salt
- pepper

preparation

1. For the vegan spaghetti, let the soy granulate soak in 300 ml of water for 10 minutes.
2. Peel the carrots and the onion and dice both very small.
3. Core the peppers and cut into small pieces.
4. Halve the olives and chop the parsley.
5. Heat the oil in a large saucepan, sauté the onion and carrots for 2 to 3 minutes.
6. Deglaze with a dash of wine (not the whole thing).
7. Add the strained tomatoes, capers, olives, the whole peeled garlic cloves, paprika and paprika powder, cinnamon, Tabasco, parsley, oregano and tomato paste and stir well.
8. Once everything is warmed up, stir in the soy granules to absorb the flavors and tomato sauce.
9. Keep adding a little of the wine until it is used up.
10. Salt and pepper everything as you like and let it simmer for 30 minutes on a low heat.
11. Stir now and then.
12. Cook the pasta in good time until al dente.

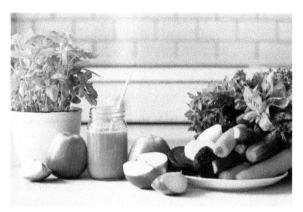

Green Easter juice

- Cooking time 15 to 30min
- Servings 4

ingredients

- 4 apples (sweet and sour)
- 3 pears
- 1 piece of ginger (the size of a thumb)
- 2 handfuls of spinach leaves (large)

preparation

1. For the Green Easter juice, first quarter the apples and pears and remove the core. Peel the ginger. Wash the spinach and spin dry.
2. Squeeze all ingredients through a juicer and collect the juice. Fill green Easter juice into glasses and serve.

Oriental spinach salad

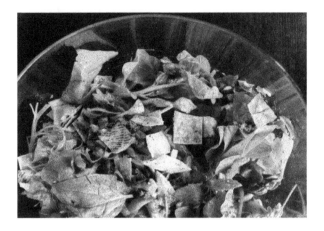

- Cooking time 30 to 60 min
- Servings 4

ingredients

- 4 handfuls of baby spinach (fresh, about 150 g)
- 1/2 onion (red)
- 6 dates (firm)
- 1/2 lemon (juice)
- 1 tbsp apple cider vinegar
- 4 tbsp olive oil
- 1/2 teaspoon cayenne pepper (or mildly spicy chili powder)
- Sea salt (to taste)
- 70 g almonds
- 2 pita breads (preferably made from whole grain)

preparation

1. To prepare, first soak the almonds overnight and peel off the skin the next morning.
2. Wash the spinach and pat dry.
3. For the dressing, finely dice half the onion and place in a salad bowl. Cut the dates into wafer-thin slices and whisk

well with the onions and the remaining dressing ingredients. Season the whole thing with salt.

4. Add the washed spinach to the dressing in the bowl.
5. For the croutons, cut the pita bread into cubes and coarsely chop the almonds. Roast both in a pan without fat for 3 to 5 minutes over medium heat.
6. To serve, mix the salad and sprinkle the croutons with the almonds on top.

Beauty summer rolls

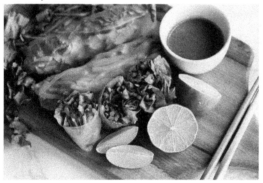

- Cooking time 30 to 60 min
- Servings 4

ingredients
- 1/4 cucumber
- 1 stick (s) celery
- 50 g red cabbage
- 50 g pineapple pulp
- 50 g avocado pulp
- 50 g baby spinach
- 2 sprig (s) of lemon balm
- 6 sheets of rice paper
- 2 tbsp soy sauce (light, light)

- 1 teaspoon tahini
- 1 teaspoon agave syrup
- 1 teaspoon lime juice
- Pepper (freshly ground)
- Turmeric (freshly ground)

preparation

1. For the beauty summer rolls, first wash the vegetables and cut them into long thin strips. Cut the pineapple and avocado into slices. Wash the spinach and shake dry. Wash the lemon balm, shake dry and pluck the leaves.
2. Soak the rice paper sheets in a large bowl of water for about 1 minute. Spread the rice paper out on a work surface. Place the vegetable strips, pineapple, lemon balm, spinach on the bottom of the rice paper sheets and fold the sides. Roll up tightly and place on a plate.
3. Mix the soy sauce, the tahini, the agave syrup, the lime juice and 2 tbsp water well and season with pepper and turmeric. Serve the sauce with the beauty summer rolls.

Peruvian parsley salad

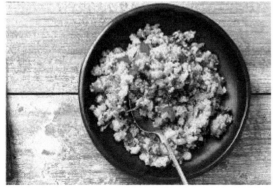

- Cooking time 30 to 60 min
- Servings 4

ingredients

- 200 g quinoa
- 400 ml of water
- 1 bunch of parsley (smooth)
- 1 bunch of mint
- 2 tomatoes (firm)
- 1/2 cucumber
- 1/2 pomegranate
- 4 tbsp olive oil
- 1/2 lemon (juice)
- Sea salt (to taste)
- Pepper (black, freshly ground, to taste)

preparation

1. For Peruvian parsley salad, first cook the quinoa in lightly salted water in a closed saucepan over medium heat for about 10 minutes, then drain.
2. Wash the parsley (with the stems), pat dry, finely chop and place in a bowl. Pluck the mint leaves from the stems and add. Cut the tomatoes (without the green parts) and the cucumber into small cubes and stir in as well. Cut the pomegranate open, carefully knock the red seeds out of one half or scrape out with a tablespoon and add to the other ingredients.
3. Fold the cooked, cooled quinoa into the salad. Drizzle with olive oil and lemon juice, season the Peruvian parsley salad with sea salt and pepper and enjoy.

Winter soup

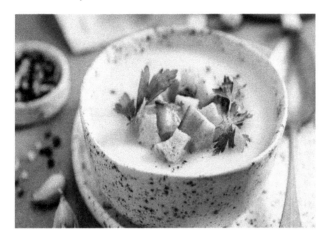

ingredients

- 150 g mung beans
- 1/2 Chinese cabbage
- 1 apple
- 2 parsley roots
- 1 onion (small)
- 1 tbsp ghee
- 1 tbsp cinnamon powder
- 1 teaspoon coriander (coarsely crushed)
- 1 pinch of clove powder
- 1 tsp black cumin
- 1/2 teaspoon pepper (coarsely crushed)
- 650 ml water (boiling)
- 30 g raisins
- 100 ml apple juice
- salt
- Sunflower sprouts (fresh)

preparation

1. For the winter soup, cut the Chinese cabbage into fine strips, cut the apple and parsley roots into cubes.
2. Finely chop the onion and garlic cloves. Heat the ghee in a saucepan, briefly roast the spices so that the cinnamon doesn't burn. Add the garlic and onion. When the scent rises, roast the vegetables for 1 to 2 minutes.
3. In the meantime, wash the soaked mung beans in a sieve, drain them and put them in the pot. Stir in and pour in the boiling water. Add the raisins and simmer covered for about 50 minutes, stirring occasionally. Add apple juice and salt. Let it steep for 5 to 10 minutes and serve the winter soup sprinkled with sunflower sprouts.

Detox Radicchio Salad

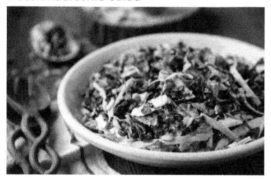

- Cooking time 15 to 30min
- Servings 4

ingredients
- 40 g radicchio (in bite-sized pieces)
- 1 orange (filleted, cut into pieces)
- 1/2 orange (juice of it)
- 2 tbsp vegetable soup
- 1 teaspoon olive oil

- salt
- Pepper (from the mill)

preparation

1. For the detox radicchio salad, prepare a salad dressing from the vegetable soup, orange juice and the olive oil. Add the radicchio and the orange and season with salt and pepper.
2. Arrange and serve the Detox Radicchio Salad.

Detox hot orange drink

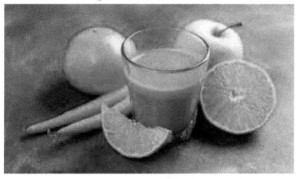

- Cooking time 30 to 60 min
- Servings 1

ingredients

- 6 pcs. Orange
- 2 sprig (s) of sage
- 3 cm ginger
- 1/2 pod (s) of chili

preparation

1. For the Detox Hot Orange Drink, first make the Detox Sud. To do this, select the sage and wash it, peel off the leaves. Wash the ginger, peel and dice if desired.

2. Put the sage and ginger in a saucepan. Cover just a little with water, bring to the boil once. Remove the stem from the chilli pepper and cut open lengthways.
3. Cut the chilli into cubes / pieces and add the chilli pepper to the brew. Let simmer for 2 minutes. Then strain and let cool down. Squeeze oranges and pour the juice into a drinking glass.
4. Add the chilli ginger brew, stir and enjoy the Detox Hot Orange drink.

Detox strawberry rose lemon water

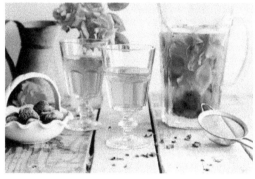

- Cooking time 30 to 60 min
- Servings 1

ingredients
- 10 strawberries (adjust quantity)
- 1/2 lemon
- 20 rose petals (not dried)
- 1500 ml water (possibly filtered)

preparation
1. For the Detox-Strawberry-Lemon Water, first prepare the strawberries (wash, remove the flower base and chop). Shake the rose petals well, but do not wash.

2. Loosen the petals liberally from the calyx. Spread out on kitchen paper and check again for any insects. Wash, dry and slice the lemon half.
3. Put the water, strawberries, lemon wedges and rose petals in a glass jug. Depending on the desired taste intensity, let the detox strawberry lemon water steep (at least two hours).

Detox blackberry lemongrass rose water

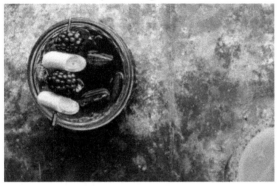

- Cooking time 30 to 60 min
- Servings 1

ingredients
- 3 tbsp blackberries
- 2 pieces of lemongrass
- Rose petals (to taste)
- 1500 ml of water

preparation
1. For the detox blackberry, lemongrass and rose water, shake the rose petals well, but do not wash. Loosen the petals liberally from the calyx.
2. Spread out on kitchen paper and check again for any insects. Sort and wash the blackberries and lemongrass.

Pound the lemongrass until soft (tin can). Put the water, blackberries and lemongrass in a carafe.

3. Finally add rose petals and stir gently once. Let it stand overnight in a cool place. Drink the detox blackberry lemongrass rose water over the next day.

Detox water

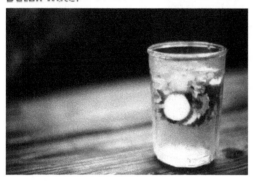

ingredients

- 2 litters of water
- 1 pc. Ginger (1 cm)
- 1 pc cucumber
- 1 piece of lemon
- 1 sprig (s) of mint (or any amount you like)

preparation

1. Carefully wash all ingredients for the detox water. Then put 2 litters of water in a large bowl. Then cut the cucumber and lemon into thin slices.

2. Put everything together in the bowl with the water and seal airtight. Put in the fridge overnight and enjoy cold the next day.

Detox multi smoothie

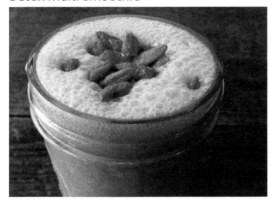

- Cooking time 30 to 60 min
- Servings 4

ingredients

- 1 pc. Clementines
- 1/2 piece of mango
- 1 piece of apples (e.g. Gala)
- 1 slice (s) of pineapple
- 1 pear
- 1 pc. Plum
- 80 ml pomegranate juice
- 10 g diced ginger
- 8 strawberries
- 1 teaspoon goji fruits
- 1/2 beetroot (cooked al dente)
- Ice cubes (to taste)

preparation

1. Prepare the fruits for the multi-detox smoothie (depending on the fruit, wash, peel, squeeze, core and chop). The clementine can also be squeezed. Soak the dried goji berries.

2. Put the fruit pieces together with the ice cubes in a juicer / blender, mix and serve immediately.

Detox strawberry lemon water

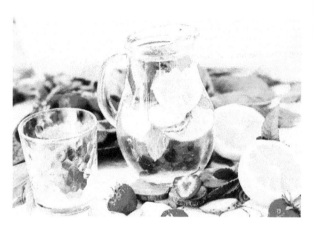

ingredients

- 10 strawberries (adjust quantity)
- 1/2 lemon
- 1 1/2 l water (possibly filtered)

preparation

1. First prepare the strawberries (wash, remove the flower base and chop).
2. Wash, dry and slice the lemon half.
3. Put the water, strawberries and lemon wedges in a glass jug.
4. Depending on the desired taste intensity, let the detox strawberry lemon water steep (at least two hours).

Detox rose flower water with lemon

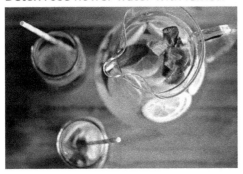

- Cooking time 30 to 60 min
- Servings 4

ingredients

- 1 handful of rose petals (unsprayed)
- 1/3 lemon (organic)
- 1 liter of water

preparation

1. First shake the rose petals well, but do not wash. Liberally loosen the petals from the calyx, otherwise it will taste bitter.
2. Spread out on kitchen paper and check again for any insects.
3. Wash, dry and slice the lemon half. Put the water and lemon wedges in a glass jug. Finally, add the rose petals and stir gently once.
4. Be sure to cover the jug so that the essential oils don't evaporate. Let it steep in the fridge overnight.
5. Drink the detox rose petal water over the next day.

Detox water with elderflower and citrus fruits

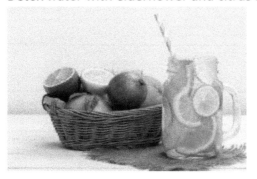

- Cooking time 30 to 60 min
- Servings 1

ingredients

- 1 l spring water (very cold, or tap water)
- 1 lemon (organic)
- 1 orange (organic)
- 2 elder flowers
- Ice cubes

preparation

1. First cut half a lemon into slices and quarter the slices. Squeeze the other half of the lemon. Do the same with the orange.
2. Put the orange and lemon slices, the orange and lemon juice, the elderflower and the ice cubes in a jug or carafe.
3. Pour on the spring water and let it steep in the refrigerator for about half an hour.

Detox pomegranate rose flower water

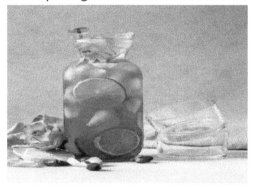

- Cooking time 30 to 60 min
- Servings 1

ingredients

- 4 tbsp pomegranate seeds
- 1 handful of rose petals (unsprayed)
- 1/3 lime (organic)
- 1250 ml of water

preparation

1. For the detox pomegranate rose petal water, shake the rose petals well, but do not wash. Liberally loosen the petals from the calyx, otherwise it will taste bitter.
2. Spread out on kitchen paper and check again for any insects. Wash, dry and slice the lime. Put the water, pomegranate seeds and lime slices in a carafe.
3. Finally add rose petals and stir gently once. Make sure to cover the carafe so that the essential oils do not evaporate. Let it stand overnight in a cool place.
4. Drink the detox pomegranate rose blossom water over the next day.

Detox summer garden smoothie

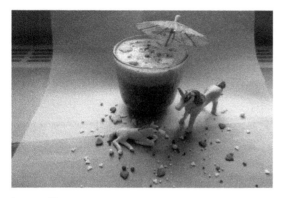

ingredients

- 20 g nettle
- 20 g baby spinach
- 1 piece of passion fruit
- 1 pc. Orange
- 1 banana
- 2 apples
- Ice cubes (to taste)
- Water (to taste)

preparation

1. Prepare the fruits and salads for the detox summer garden smoothie (depending on the type, sort, wash, peel, squeeze, core and chop - depending on the mixer power).

2. Put everything together in a blender and puree until the desired consistency is achieved. Depending on the amount of water, the smoothie will be thicker or thinner.

Detox drink strawberry rose

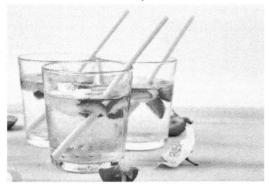

- Cooking time 15 to 30 min

ingredients

- 2 pears (e.g., Williams Christ)
- 100 ml pomegranate juice
- 12 strawberries
- 1 tbsp goji berries
- 2 tbsp rose water
- 1 teaspoon lime juice
- 1 pinch of cinnamon
- Ice cubes (to taste)

preparation

1. Prepare the fruits for the Detox Drink Strawberry-Rose (depending on the fruit, wash, remove the flower base, peel, core and chop). Soak the goji berries in a little water and let them drain.
2. Put the fruits and remaining ingredients in a blender with the ice cubes, mix and serve immediately.

Mango and chilli detox drink

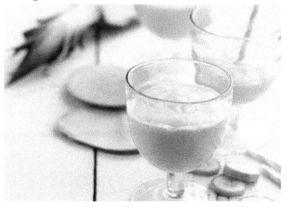

- Cooking time 15 to 30 min

ingredients

- 2 pieces of mangos (fully ripe)
- 1/2 lime (juice of it)
- Chili peppers (to taste)
- 1/2 pc. Organic orange (zest of it)

preparation

1. For the mango-chili detox drink, first wash the mango, peel it and cut out the stone. Chop the mango into small pieces depending on the juicing power.
2. Wash and drain the chilli pepper and remove the stem and partitions. Juice the mango and chilli and mix with the other ingredients.
3. Pour the drink into a jug and dilute with water as desired. Serve the mango-chili detox drink chilled.

Radish soup detox

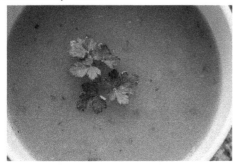

ingredients

- 1 teaspoon oil
- 1 bunch of radishes
- 1 stalk of celery
- 500 ml of water
- 2 carrots (small)
- 1/2 teaspoon herb salt
- 1/2 piece of soup cubes (vegan)

preparation

1. For the radish soup, heat the oil, chop the carrot and fry in the oil. Chop the radishes and add them.
2. Also cut the celery into narrow strips, sauté, pour water on top and season. Let cook for about 10 minutes.

Autumn smoothie detox

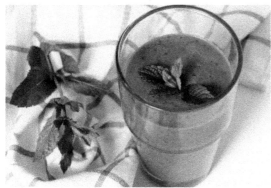

- Cooking time 5 to 15 min
- Servings 1

ingredients

- 1/8 head red cabbage
- 2 apples
- 2 tbsp Powidl

preparation

1. For the autumn smoothie, cut out one eighth of the red cabbage, use the remaining cabbage for other purposes. Cut away the stalk from the red cabbage wedge.
2. Core the apples, the skin can stay on. Smooth the red cabbage and apples finely in the smoothie maker, add the Powidl and drink the drink quickly.

Wild garlic soup with daisies

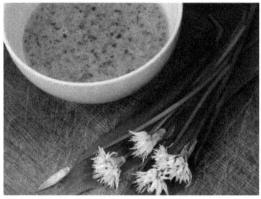

- Cooking time 30 to 60 min
- Servings 4

ingredients

- 1 tbsp butter
- 1 onion
- 2 cloves of garlic

- 100 ml white wine (dry)
- 50 ml Noilly Prat
- 500 ml clear soup
- 300 ml whipped cream
- 20 grams of flour
- 20 g butter
- 1 squirt of lemon juice
- salt
- Pepper (freshly ground)
- 4 tbsp wild garlic paste
- 50 g parsley leaves
- 150 g wild garlic
- approx. 150 ml sunflower oil
- about 1 teaspoon of salt
- 1 handful of daisies

preparation

1. For the wild garlic soup with daisies, first prepare the wild garlic paste: Blanch the parsley and wild garlic in salted water (scalded) and rinse in ice water so that the beautiful green colour is retained. Express well. Mix with sunflower oil and salt.
2. For the flour butter, knead 20 g flour and 20 g butter well. Let rest in the fridge.
3. Finely chop the onion and garlic. Heat the butter in a saucepan and roast the onions until golden. Add garlic and briefly toast, then deglaze with white wine and Noilly Prat. Pour in the soup and cream. Thicken with the flour butter and simmer the soup for 15-20 minutes over low heat.
4. Stir in 4 tbsp wild garlic paste and season with salt, pepper and a squeeze of lemon juice.

5. The wild garlic soup into soup plates and garnish decorate with daisies.

Asparagus and wild garlic soup

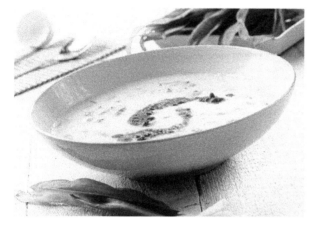

ingredients

- 500 g asparagus (white)
- 2 handfuls of wild garlic
- 200 ml whipped cream
- 1 teaspoon lemon juice
- 1 pinch of sugar
- 3 tbsp butter (ice cold)
- salt
- Pepper (freshly ground)
- 1 liter of vegetable soup or asparagus cooking water

preparation

1. For the asparagus and wild garlic soup , peel the asparagus stalks starting at the head end and remove the woody asparagus ends. Let the bowls boil with a pinch of sugar in 1 liter of salted water for 10 minutes. Strain and bring the brew to the boil again.
2. Rinse the wild garlic leaves with cold water and roughly chop. Cut the asparagus spears into pieces. First cook the

asparagus tips in the asparagus stock for about 5 minutes and then lift them out. Now put in the asparagus pieces and the wild garlic and cook for about 12 minutes. Stir in the cream towards the end of the cooking time. Remove from the heat and puree with the hand blender.

3. Stir in the ice-cold butter in flakes and season the soup with salt, pepper and a little lemon juice. Place the asparagus tips in the asparagus and wild garlic soup before serving.

Green asparagus soup

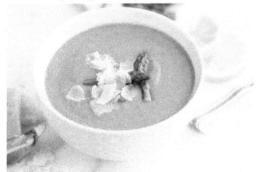

ingredients

- 700 g asparagus (green)
- 300 g asparagus (white)
- 300 g potatoes
- 1 apple
- 1000 ml of vegetable soup
- 150 g crème fraîche
- salt
- Pepper (freshly ground)

preparation

1. Thinly peel the white asparagus in the lower third of the stalks from top to bottom. The green asparagus does not have to be peeled. Cut the lower ends small (completely cut

away woody areas). Wash and drain both types of asparagus.

2. Cut the asparagus into pieces, put the heads to one side. Rinse and peel the potatoes and apples, remove the core from the apple and cut both into pieces.

3. Boil up the vegetable soup and cook the pieces of vegetables and apples in it for 20 minutes at a low temperature with the lid on.

4. Puree the soup, fold in the crème fraîche, sauté the asparagus heads for 8 minutes at a low temperature.

5. Season the asparagus soup well with salt and freshly ground pepper.

Woodruff asparagus soup

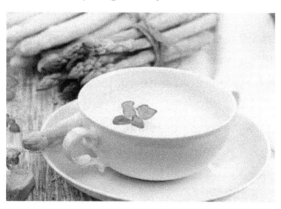

ingredients
- 600 g asparagus (white)
- 1 twig (s) woodruff (slightly withered)
- 1 pinch of sugar
- some salt
- Olive oil (for frying)
- 1 onion

- 80 g potatoes
- 120 ml whipped cream
- some pepper (freshly ground)
- some nutmeg
- 1 squirt of lemon juice

preparation

1. For the woodruff asparagus soup, first peel the asparagus and cut off about 2 cm at the bottom. Cut the rest into bite-sized pieces. Pick up the shells. Peel and finely dice the onion. Peel the potatoes and dice them too.
2. Boil about a liter of water with the asparagus peels, the woodruff, sugar and salt. Then turn off the stove and let the brew stand for about 10 minutes. Then empty through a sieve.
3. Sweat the onions in a little oil. Add the asparagus and potatoes. Deglaze with the stock and add the whipped cream. Put the lid on and simmer for about 20 minutes. Then season with freshly grated nutmeg, lemon juice, salt and pepper.
4. The Woodruff asparagus soup puree and serve.

Pasta with artichokes and prawns

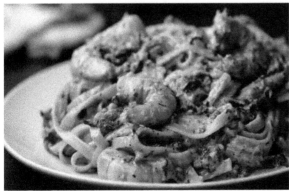

- Cooking time 30 to 60 min
- Servings 4

ingredients

- 400 g pasta (of your choice, e.g., penne, spaghetti, farfalle)
- 16 Quality First frozen king prawns (shell less, defrosted)
- 25 g Quality First frozen onions (defrosted)
- 200 g Quality First pickled artichokes
- 200 ml whipped cream
- 2 tbsp Quality First rapeseed oil
- 4 tbsp Quality First balsamic vinegar
- 25 g Quality First Italian herbs
- 1 parmesan cheese (small)
- salt
- pepper

preparation

1. Cook the pasta according to the packet's instructions in plenty of salted water until al dente and drain.
2. While the pasta is cooking, prepare the sauce: quarter the artichokes. Heat the rapeseed oil in a pan and fry the onions, prawns and artichokes. Deglaze with the vinegar and that
3. Stir in the cream, reduce slightly. Add the pasta and the Italian herbs, stir briefly and season well with salt and pepper.
4. Arrange in deep plates and sprinkle the pasta with artichokes and prawns with freshly grated or grated Parmesan to taste.

Spelled penne with grapes and strips of chicken

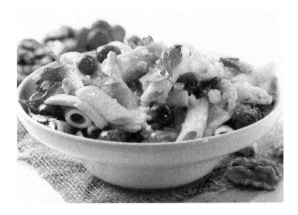

ingredients

- 450 g rake ice cream spelled penne
- 1 chicken breast
- 1 shallot
- 20 grapes (red, seedless)
- 50 ml white wine
- 150 ml whipped cream
- 2 tbsp walnuts (chopped)
- 1/2 bunch of parsley
- Sunflower oil
- salt
- pepper

preparation

1. The spelled penne with grapes and strips of chicken, first peel the shallot and cut into small cubes, then the chicken breast into thin strips.
2. Boil the pasta in plenty of salted water until al dente, drain and set aside.
3. Sear shallots, grapes and chicken strips with a little sunflower oil on all sides. Remove from the pan, deglaze the

roasting residue with white wine, pour in the whipped cream and reduce slightly.

4. Add the chicken strips and grapes again and let simmer a little more. Before serving, stir the parsley leaves and walnuts into the spelled penne with grapes and strips of chicken and season with salt and pepper

Spelled Dralli with baby spinach and coconut

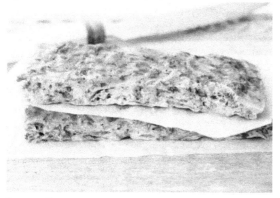

ingredients

- 400 g Recheis Naturgenuss Spelled Dralli
- 2 shallots
- 2 cm ginger root
- 1/4 pod (s) of chilli
- 200 ml coconut milk
- 100 g baby spinach leaves
- 1/2 lime (organic, zest and juice)
- 3 tbsp sunflower oil
- salt
- pepper

preparation

1. For the spelled twist with baby spinach and coconut, peel shallots and ginger and cut into small cubes, core and finely chop the chilli pepper. Rinse the spinach with cold water.

2. Cook the spelled twist according to the instructions on the package, pour it off and set aside.
3. Fry shallots in oil until translucent, add twisted sauce and pour coconut milk on top. Season with chilli, ginger, lime juice and zest and season with salt and pepper.
4. Add the spinach leaves, remove the pan from the heat and toss it through once so that the spinach leaves collapse. The Dinkel Dralli with baby spinach and coconut distribute soup plates and serve immediately.

Tagliatelle with shrimp

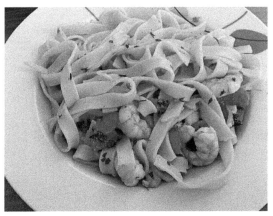

ingredients
- 220 g tagliatelle
- 1 clove (s) of garlic
- 1 tbsp olive oil
- 150 g shrimp
- 150 g Bresso traditional fine herbs (1 cup)
- 30 g whipped cream
- 1/16 l milk
- pepper
- salt

- Basil (fresh)

preparation

1. For the tagliatelle with shrimp, cook the tagliatelle al dente. In a pan, sauté the finely chopped garlic in olive oil. Add the shrimp and fry.

2. Stir in Bresso traditional fine herbs, cream and milk and bring to the boil briefly. Season to taste with salt and freshly ground pepper.

3. Add to the tagliatelle, mix well and serve on preheated plates. Sprinkle fresh, chopped basil generously on top and serve immediately.

Tagliatelle with zucchini and fennel vegetables

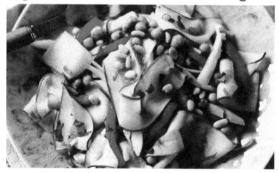

- Cooking time 60 min
- Servings 4

ingredients

For the pasta dough:

- 250 g Fini's finest pasta semolina
- 2 eggs (M)
- 1/2 teaspoon salt
- 2 tbsp olive oil
- 4 tbsp water

For the vegetables:

- 1 tuber (s) of fennel
- 1 zucchini (yellow, small)
- 2 shallots
- 1 clove of garlic
- 1/2 teaspoon fennel seeds
- some lemon zest (organic)
- 50 ml lemon juice
- 150 g crème fraiche

Furthermore:
- 100 g flaked almonds
- salt
- pepper
- 100 g pecorino cheese
- Olive oil (for frying)
- Cress (for garnish)

preparation

1. For the tagliatelle with zucchini-fennel-vegetables, first combine all the pasta dough ingredients in a bowl and knead into a smooth dough. Wrap the dough in cling film and let rest for about 20 minutes.
2. Briefly toast the almond flakes without oil.
3. Roll out pasta dough thinly on a floured work surface. Flour both sides well, roll up the plate. Cut the strips to the desired width. Let the pasta dry a little on a tray dusted with flour and loosen it up to stick together.
4. Peel and roughly grate the fennel and zucchini. Put the fennel greens aside. Finely chop the shallots and garlic.
5. Bring water to a boil with 1 teaspoon salt in a large saucepan.
6. Heat the olive oil, fry the shallots and garlic. Add the fennel, zucchini grated, fennel seeds, lemon peel, and fry for 3-4

minutes. Deglaze with lemon juice. Remove from the stove and stir in the creme fraiche. Salt and pepper.

7. Put the pasta in the boiling water and cook for 2-3 minutes until al dente. Strain and add to the vegetables with 2-3 tablespoons of cooking water. Chop the fennel greens and stir in. The tagliatelle with zucchini and fennel arranges on the plates and serve sprinkled with flaked almonds, watercress and pecorino.

Poppy seed cake baked in the cup

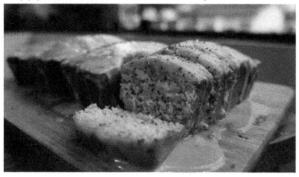

- Cooking time 60 min
- Servings 6

Ingredients

- 4 eggs
- 90 g of sugar
- 1 pinch of salt
- 50 g butter (liquid)
- 125 g poppy seeds (ground)
- Butter (to spread the cups)
- Granulated sugar (for sprinkling the cups)
- Icing sugar (for sprinkling)

preparation

1. Separate the eggs for the poppy seed cake . Beat egg whites together with 1/3 of the sugar and salt until stiff.
2. Beat the yolks together with the remaining sugar until frothy and stir in the poppy seeds and melted butter.
3. Then fold in the egg whites. Preheat the oven to 170 degrees. Spread the butter and granulated sugar over small fireproof cups or molds and sprinkle them on top.
4. Pour in the poppy seed mixture, place the cups on a baking sheet and bake for about 20 minutes. Sprinkle with icing sugar while it is still warm and serve the poppy seed cake immediately.

Pomegranate granite

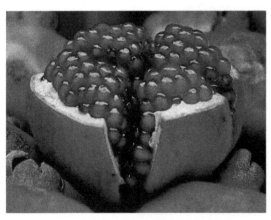

- Cooking time 60 min
- Servings 4

ingredients

- 2 pcs. Blood oranges
- 2 pieces of limes
- 5 pcs. Pomegranates
- 200 g Brunch Légere classic

- 75 g sugar
- 1 packet of vanilla sugar
- Mint (or waffles for garnish)

preparation

1. For the pomegranate granite, squeeze blood oranges and limes. Halve the pomegranates and also use a citrus press to extract the juice. Beat the blood orange, lime and pomegranate juice and brunch vigorously with the hand mixer. Season to taste with sugar and vanilla sugar.
2. Place in a metal bowl and let freeze in the freezer for about 6 hours. Take out the granite and roughly chop it with a spoon handle.
3. Put the pomegranate granité in very well chilled glasses, garnish with mint and small waffles if you like and serve immediately.

Berry tartlets with vanilla cream

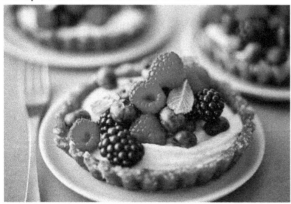

- Cooking time 30 to 60 min
- Servings 4

ingredients

- Butter (for the molds)

- 4 tbsp raspberry jam (other type to taste)
- 100 g blueberries
- 100 g raspberries
- 1 handful of blackberries
- 1 handful of strawberries
- 1 sprig (s) of mint

For the cake bases:
- 300 g of flour
- 200 g butter (room temperature)
- 1 egg yolk
- 100 g icing sugar
- 1 pinch of salt

For the cream:
- 1 packet of custard powder
- 500 ml of milk
- 2 tbsp sugar
- 200 g mascarpone
- 1 pod of vanilla (scraped pulp)
- 1/2 teaspoon tonka bean (grated)

preparation

1. For the cake bases, knead a shortcrust pastry from the ingredients listed. Wrap the dough ball in cling film and leave to rest in the refrigerator for about 20 minutes.
2. In the meantime, cook a pudding for the cream of pudding powder, milk and sugar according to the package instructions. Immediately cover the surface with cling film and let the pudding cool.
3. Preheat the oven to 200 ° C. Grease the tartlet molds.
4. Roll out the dough about 5 mm thick on a floured work surface and line the molds with it, cutting off the protruding

edges. Prick the bases several times with a fork and bake in the hot oven for about 10 minutes until golden brown.

5. Let the cake bases cool for a few minutes in the molds, then carefully remove and let cool down completely on a baking rack.

6. To finish the cream, mix the mascarpone, vanilla pulp and tonka bean. Mix the cooled vanilla pudding with the hand mixer until smooth, add the mascarpone mixture and mix everything into a smooth cream.

7. Wash and sort the berries and remove the stems as necessary.

8. Brush the cooled cake bases with jam and distribute the cream evenly over it. Cover with the berries decoratively and garnish with mint to taste and serve.

Strawberry yogurt tart

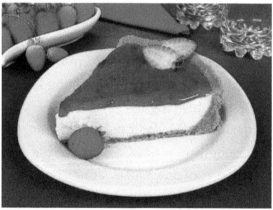

ingredients

For the shortcrust pastry:

- 250 g of flour
- 2 tbsp sugar
- 1 pinch of salt
- 1 packet of vanillin sugar

- 125 ml vegetable oil (neutral)
- 3 teaspoons of skimmed milk yogurt

For the filling:

- 2 tbsp sugar
- 3 sheets of gelatin
- 1/2 lemon (untreated)
- 1 tbsp fine sugar
- 250 ml of yogurt
- 1/2 pod (s) vanilla (pulp)

preparation

1. For the shortcrust pastry, mix the sugar, flour, vanilla sugar and salt. Quickly mix in the oil and yoghurt and knead to a smooth dough.
2. Cool the shortcrust pastry wrapped in foil for 1/2 hour. Preheat the oven to 200 ° C. Roll out the dough thinly and use it to spread a fruit cake tin. Prick the bottom with a fork and bake the dough for about 10 to 15 minutes. Let cool down.
3. Rinse and dry the strawberries. Soak the gelatine in cold tap water for 5 minutes, squeeze it out, heat it with the lemon juice in a saucepan and dissolve it.
4. Mix the yoghurt with the vanilla pod's pulp and stir in the liquid gelatine, tablespoon at a time. Remove from the kitchen stove, stir and let cool down lukewarm.
5. Pour onto the finished shortcrust pastry and distribute the whole berries on top. Peel the lemon skin in a spiral shape and cover with it.
6. Dust the cake with fine sugar for serving.

Berry millefeuille with curd cream

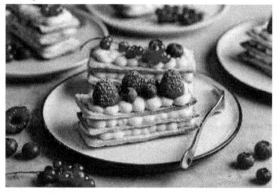

ingredients

- 1 packet of strudel pastry sheets
- 40 g butter (liquid)
- 50 g poppy seeds (ground)
- Icing sugar (for sprinkling)
- 250 g raspberries
- Lemon balm

For the curd cream:

- 250 g curd cheese
- 100 g yogurt
- 100 g icing sugar
- 1 teaspoon vanilla sugar
- 50 g poppy seeds (ground)
- 1 lemon (untreated, juice and zest)
- 250 ml whipped cream

preparation

1. For the berry millefeuille with curd cream, first preheat the oven to 200 ° C top / bottom heat.
2. Stir the curd cheese with yogurt, icing sugar, vanilla sugar, poppy seeds, lemon juice and zest until smooth. Beat the

whipped cream until stiff and fold into the curd cream. Refrigerate.

3. Roll up the strudel pastry, brush with melted butter and sprinkle with poppy seeds and icing sugar. Bake in the oven for about 5 minutes until crispy. Let cool down.
4. Wash and drain raspberries.
5. Spread some curd cream on plates, break off a piece of the strudel dough and place on top. Spread a little more curd cream and a few raspberries on top and repeat this process three to four times until you get a little tower. Serve the berry millefeuille with curd cream, garnished with fresh raspberries and fresh lemon balm.

Raspberry yogurt mousse

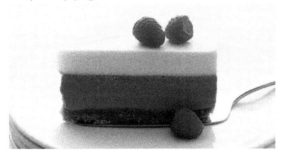

- Cooking time 30 to 60 min
- Servings 4

ingredients

For the raspberry mousse:
- 100 g raspberries (strained)
- 0.5 lemon (squeezed juice)
- 130 g Guma pâtisserie cream
- 40 g icing sugar

For the yogurt mousse:
- 100 g natural yogurt

- 0.5 lemon (squeezed juice)
- 40 g icing sugar
- 130 g Guma pâtisserie cream
- 1 egg white
- 15 g granulated sugar

preparation

1. For the raspberry yoghurt mousse, pre-cool the glasses in the refrigerator. For the yoghurt mousse, beat the egg white and granulated sugar into snow.
2. For the raspberry mousse, whip up the Guma Pâtisserie Cream until it has a firm but airy consistency.
3. Mix in the raspberries, lemon juice and icing sugar. Pour the mixture into the glasses and put in a cool place.
4. For the yoghurt mousse, whip the Guma pâtisserie cream until it has a firm but still airy consistency.
5. Mix in the yogurt, lemon juice and icing sugar and fold in the egg whites. Arrange on the raspberry mousse so that 2 nice layers are created.
6. The raspberry yogurt mousse refrigerates for at least 6 hours in the refrigerator.

Pasta salad with pesto Genovese

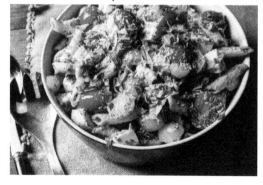

- Cooking time 15 to 30 min

- servings 4

ingredients

- 300 g Farfalle
- 50 g rocket
- 200 g cherry tomatoes
- pepper
- 80 g bresaola
- 10 ml of vegetable soup
- 5 ml white wine vinegar
- 3 tbsp Barilla Pesto Genovese
- 3-4 tbsp olive oil

preparation

1. Bring plenty of salted water to the boil for the pasta salad. Add the farfalle and cook until al dente. Pour into a sieve and rinse briefly in cold water to prevent the pasta from sticking.
2. While the farfalle is cooking, wash the arugula and drain well.
3. Halve the cherry tomatoes and season the cut surfaces with salt and pepper. Let it steep briefly.
4. Cut the bresaola or into narrow strips. In a large bowl, mix the bouillon, vinegar, pesto Genovese, salt and pepper together and then add the olive oil.
5. Before serving, add the Farfalle, rocket and cherry tomatoes to the sauce and mix everything carefully. Season if necessary.
6. Garnish the pasta salad with the bresaola

vegetable soup

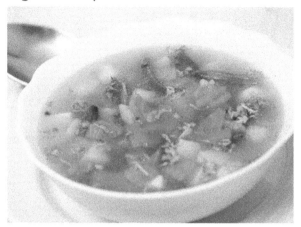

- Cooking time 30 to 60 min
- servings 4

ingredients

- 1 pc onion (small)
- Some oil
- 200 g carrots
- 100 g parsnips
- 100 g peas
- parsley
- 200 g potatoes
- 1000 ml of water
- salt

preparation

1. For the vegetable soup, fry the finely chopped onion in a little oil until translucent. Cut the carrots and parsnips into small pieces and roast them well. Chop the parsley and fry briefly.
2. Add the frozen peas, season with salt. Pour water on. Cut the potatoes into small cubes and add. Cook until soft.

Potato and vegetable soup with Black Forest ham

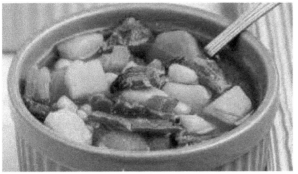

- Cooking time 30 to 60 min
- Servings 4

ingredients

- 2 onions (small, white, peeled)
- 2 cloves of garlic (peeled)
- 1 carrot (peeled)
- 1 turnip (yellow, peeled)
- 1/4 celery (peeled)
- 1/4 stick (s) leek
- 100 g Black Forest ham (sliced)
- 1 pinch of saffron
- 1 bay leaf
- 1 liter of vegetable soup
- 10 g porcini mushrooms (dried)
- 1/2 teaspoon thyme (dried)
- 1/2 teaspoon caraway seeds (ground)
- 500 g potatoes (raw, peeled)
- 200 ml whipped cream
- salt
- pepper
- Sunflower oil

preparation

1. For the potato and vegetable soup with Black Forest ham, first cut the onion, garlic, carrot, yellow beet, celery and leek into fine cubes. Cut the Black Forest ham into fine strips.

2. Lightly toast the ham in a little oil. Add onion and garlic and roast colourless. Add the root vegetables and roast briefly. Add saffron and bay leaf and pour on the soup.

3. Soak the porcini mushrooms in a little lukewarm water for about 5 minutes, chop them finely and add to the soup with the soaking liquid. Season with thyme, caraway seeds, salt and pepper.

4. Cut the potatoes into cubes approx. 1 x 1 cm and cook them in the soup for about 10-15 minutes. Season the soup to taste and remove the bay leaf.

5. Add half of the whipped cream to the soup. Beat the other half and garnish the potato and vegetable soup with Black Forest ham with it.

Vegetable soup for the AND SOY Maker

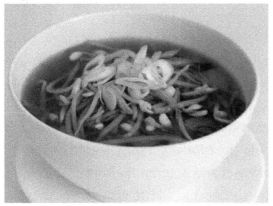

ingredients

- 200 g potatoes
- 100 g carrots
- 100 g yellow beets
- 100 g zucchini
- Vegetable soup (clear)
- 1 tbsp olive oil
- salt
- pepper

preparation

1. For the vegetable soup, first cut the vegetables into large cubes. Put the diced vegetables, salt, pepper and olive oil in the AND SOY Maker and fill up with clear vegetable soup (total amount between the two marks).

2. Close the AND SOY, turn it up and select program 2. The vegetable soup is ready after about 30 minutes. Then season again to taste.

Stew with spring vegetables and wild garlic pesto

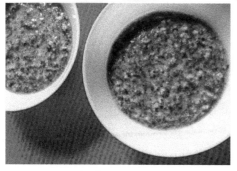

- Cooking time 30 to 60 min
- Servings 4

ingredients

For the stew:

- 8 carrots (small, young)
- 100 g snow peas
- 1 kohlrabi
- 150 g peas
- 100 g rhubarb
- 3 radishes
- 1 stick (s) spring onions
- 1 stick (s) celery (green)
- 500 ml of vegetable soup
- salt
- pepper

For the pesto:

- 200 g wild garlic
- 1 bunch of basil
- 50 g pine nuts
- 30 g parmesan (freshly grated)
- 100 ml of olive oil

- salt
- pepper

preparation

1. For the pesto, cut the wild garlic (and if the wild garlic is too hot, add a bunch of basil) into large pieces.
2. Roast the pine nuts in a pan without oil until golden, do not puree all ingredients in a food processor or with a mortar, add the olive oil, season with salt and pepper.
3. Peel the carrots and cut into small cubes, strips or pieces, cut the radishes into quarters, the rhubarb and celery small cubes, halve the snow peas, cut the spring onions into fine rings.
4. Cover the carrots, radishes with the soup and simmer for 5-8 minutes. Add the remaining ingredients and simmer for another 5 minutes. Add the pesto and season to taste with salt and pepper.
5. Arrange the stew in a deep plate and garnish with a little basil.

Radish Soup

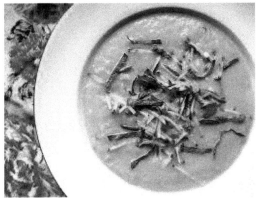

- Cooking time 30 to 60 min
- Servings 4

ingredients

- 300 g potatoes
- 1 onion (medium)
- 2 bunch of radishes
- 2 tbsp olive oil
- 375 ml of vegetable soup
- 200 g sour cream (or crème fraîche)
- salt
- pepper
- nutmeg
- Cress (for garnish)

preparation

1. Peel the potatoes and cut into small cubes. Peel onion and chop finely. Rinse the radishes well, coarsely chop two thirds of the leaves. Cut the radishes into thin slices (and cut them in half if necessary).
2. Heat the oil in a saucepan and sauté the onion and the chopped radish leaves. Add the potatoes and the soup. Cook everything for about 15 minutes in a closed saucepan.
3. Puree the soup with the hand blender. Add the sour cream or crème fraîche. Let the soup boil briefly and season with the spices.
4. Add the radish slices to the radish soup.
5. Fill into plates or soup bowls and garnish with a dollop of crème fraîche or sour cream and the cress.

Potato soup with prawns

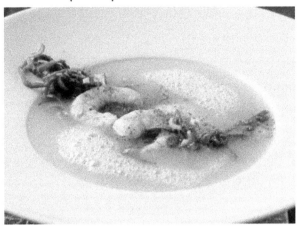

ingredients

- 500 g potatoes (floury, peeled, diced)
- 2 onions (finely chopped)
- 1 tbsp curry (mild)
- 2 tbsp clarified butter
- 750 ml of vegetable soup
- 225 g leek (cut into fine rings)
- salt
- Pepper (freshly ground)
- 250 g prawns
- 100 ml of milk
- 100 ml whipped cream

preparation

1. For the potato soup with prawns, first sauté the potatoes, onions and curry in hot clarified butter while stirring.
2. Pour in the soup and cover and cook for about 15 minutes.

3. Puree the soup with the hand blender and season with salt, pepper and possibly more curry.
4. Add the prawns, leek and milk and bring to the boil once. Stir in the whipped cream and season again to taste.
5. The potato soup with shrimp pollinates for serving with some curry.

Potato and mushroom soup with raw ham chips

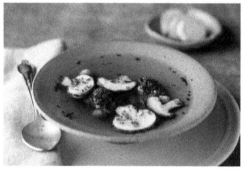

- Cooking time 30 to 60 min
- Servings 4

ingredients
- 50 g butter
- 100 g onions (finely chopped)
- 20 grams of flour
- 1 tbsp marjoram
- 1 l vegetable soup (or water)
- 500 g potatoes (floury; cut into small cubes)
- 1 packet of mushroom brunch
- salt
- Pepper (from the mill)
- 4 sheets of raw ham (cut)

preparation

1. For the potato and mushroom soup, melt the butter in a pan and brown the onion in it, add the flour and marjoram and roast briefly.
2. Pour in the soup or water, stir in the brunch and add the potatoes.
3. Simmer for about 30 minutes and season with salt and pepper.
4. Carefully place the raw ham on baking paper and bake in the oven at 180 ° C for about 10 minutes. Take out, let cool down and only take off the baking sheet when it is cold.
5. Then serve the raw ham chips in the hot potato and mushroom soup.

Vegan raspberry tartlets

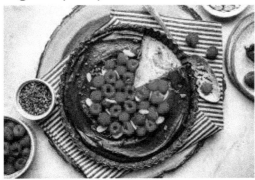

Preparation: 1 h 45 min

Ingredients

- 150 g delicate oat flakes
- 100 g spelled flour type 1050
- 90 g solid coconut oil
- 2 ½ tbsp rice syrup
- 375 g soy curd

- ½ vanilla pod
- 1 pinch organic lemon peel
- 1 stem mint
- 75 g raspberries

Preparation steps

1. Put the oat flakes and spelled flour in a bowl, add coconut oil, 1.5 tbsp rice syrup and quickly crumble everything with your hands. If necessary, add 1–2 tablespoons of cold water so that the shortcrust dough does not get too dry. Line 6 tartlet molds with the dough, prick the bases several times with a fork and bake in a preheated oven at 180 ° C (fan oven: 160 ° C; gas: level 3) for 7-10 minutes.
2. In the meantime, mix the soy quark with 1 tbsp rice syrup. Halve the vanilla pod lengthways, scrape out the pulp and add to the soy quark. Also add lemon zest and stir the quark mixture until smooth.
3. Take the tartlets out of the oven and let them cool for 5 minutes. Wash the mint, shake dry and pick off the leaves. Spread the quark on the tartlets, decorate with mint and raspberries and serve.

Blueberry yogurt shake

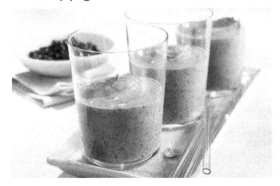

- Preparation: 10 min

ingredients

- 600 g yogurt (3.5% fat)
- 1 banana
- 100 ml milk (3.5% fat)
- 1 pinch vanilla powder
- 150 g fresh blueberries
- 50 g frozen raspberries
- 2 tbsp chia seeds

Preparation steps

1. Add yogurt, banana, 100 ml milk and vanilla powder to a blender and puree. Pour 1/3 of the shake into a container and set aside.
2. Wash the blueberries and drain them in a colander. Add 120 g blueberries to the rest of the shake in the blender along with the raspberries and chia seeds and puree them finely.
3. Divide the blueberry shake between 4 glasses or screw-top bottles. Spread the yogurt shake on top. Serve garnished with the rest of the blueberries or close the bottle and take away.

Fruit soup

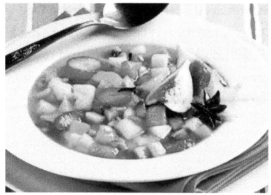

- Preparation: 35 min

ingredients

- 150 g raspberries
- 150 g strawberries
- 2 oranges
- 1 ripe pear
- 1 little apple
- 60 g roasted white almond nuts
- 4 tbsp lemon juice
- 4 tbsp whole cane sugar
- 100 ml apple juice not from concentrate
- 50 ml cranberry juice mother juice
- 250 ml water

Preparation steps

1. Sort the raspberries. Clean, wash and cut the strawberries in half. Wash the pear, cut in half, core and cut into fine wedges. Thoroughly peel and fillet the oranges. Peel the apple and cut into small cubes.

2. Caramelize the whole cane sugar in a saucepan and deglaze with apple juice, cranberry juice and water, then simmer until the sugar has dissolved. Remove the saucepan from the stove and add the fruit to the hot liquid and lemon juice.
3. Mix in the almonds, let cool, then serve lukewarm or cold. A dollop of yogurt or whipped cream goes well with the fruit soup.

Pumpkin cream soup with hazelnuts

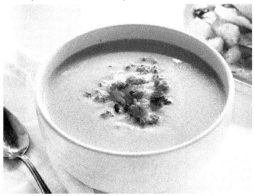

- Preparation: 40 min
- cooking time 1 h
- servings 4

ingredients
- 800 g nutmeg pumpkin
- ½ rod leek
- ½ rod celery
- 2 branches rosemary
- 2 tbsp olive oil
- salt
- pepper
- 4 juniper berries

- 250 ml non-alcoholic beer
- 500 ml vegetable broth
- 80 g hazelnut kernels
- 30 g butter (2 tbsp)
- 50 g whipped cream
- 180 g greek yogurt
- chilli flakes

Preparation steps

1. Peel the pumpkin, remove the seeds and fibers and cut the flesh into small pieces. Clean, wash and chop the leek and celery. Wash rosemary, shake dry and finely chop needles.
2. Heat oil in a pot. Sauté the prepared ingredients for 6–8 minutes over medium heat. Season with salt and pepper, add the juniper berries and deglaze with beer. Reduce the liquid by half in about 10 minutes. Pour in the vegetable stock and simmer the soup for 25 minutes over low heat.
3. In the meantime, toast the hazelnuts in the butter over medium heat for 3 minutes. Then take it off the stove.
4. Puree the soup with the cream, then strain with a spoon through a fine sieve into a saucepan and season to taste. Spread the soup on bowls, drizzle with yogurt and sprinkle with hazelnuts and chilli flakes.

Celery and pumpkin soup

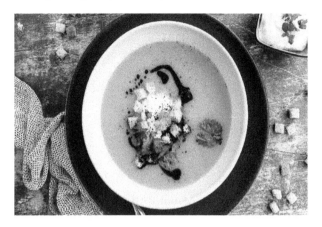

ingredients

- 1 shallot
- 20 g ginger (1 piece)
- 400 g celeriac (1 piece)
- 400 g hokkaido pumpkin (1 piece)
- 1 tbsp olive oil
- 1 l vegetable broth
- 1 tsp turmeric powder
- ½ tsp curry powder
- salt
- pepper
- chilli flakes
- 1 branch thyme

Preparation steps

1. Peel the shallot, ginger and celery and cut into small cubes. Clean the pumpkin, wash, cut in half, remove the seeds and cut the pulp into small cubes.
2. Heat oil in a saucepan. Sauté shallot and ginger in it for 2 minutes over medium heat. Add vegetables and sauté for 5

minutes. Pour in the broth, add turmeric and curry, season with salt and pepper and simmer over medium heat for about 20 minutes.

3. In the meantime, wash the thyme, shake dry and pick off the leaves.

4. Finely puree the soup with a hand blender and season with salt and pepper. Distribute the soup in soup bowls and garnish with crushed pepper, chilli flakes and thyme leaves.

Quick beetroot drink with chives

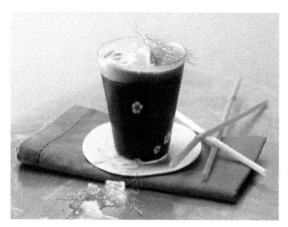

ingredients
- 50 g onions
- 1 clove of garlic

- 150 ml beetroot juice
- 50 ml carrot juice
- 3 chives
- ice cubes

Preparation steps

1. Peel the onion and garlic. Cut the onion into pieces and squeeze it over a glass with a garlic press.
2. Squeeze in the garlic, stir in the beetroot and carrot juice well. Add ice cubes. Wash the chives, shake dry and garnish the drink with them.

Mini cheesecak with blueberries

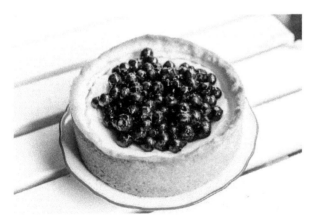

- Preparation: 30 min
- cooking time 2 h 30 min
- servings 4

ingredients

- 6 spelled ladyfingers without sugar crust
- 2 tbsp lemon juice
- 1 sheet white gelatin
- 4 tbsp blueberries
- 1 pinch bourbon vanilla powder
- 40 g cream cheese (2 tbsp)
- 80 g low-fat quark (4 tbsp)
- 1 tbsp whole cane sugar
- 30 g whipped cream (3 el)
- 20 g chopped pistachios (2 tbsp)

Preparation steps

1. Roughly chop the sponge fingers and fill into 4 glasses. Drizzle with a little lemon juice.
2. Wash the blueberries, sort, clean, drain well, mix with the vanilla powder, and let it be steep for 20 minutes.
3. Soak the gelatine in cold water. Mix the cream cheese with the quark and whole cane sugar, dissolve the gelatine dripping wet in a saucepan over low heat (do not boil!) And stir in 2 tablespoons of the cheese mixture. Pour the mixture back to the rest of the mass, stir until smooth and fold in the whipped cream.
4. Finally, mix in the blueberries and pour the mixture on the ladyfingers. Sprinkle with chopped pistachios and put in the fridge for 2 hours. Garnish each cheesecake with a heart biscuit and serve immediately.

Cress cocktail with cucumber

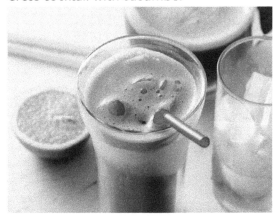

- Preparation: 10 min

ingredients
- 1 box garden cress
- 350 g cucumber
- 100 ml celery juice
- ice cubes

Preparation steps
1. Cut the cress leaves from the bed with kitchen scissors and set about 1 teaspoon aside. Put the rest in a blender.
2. Clean and peel the cucumber, cut a thick slice and roughly dice the rest.
3. Puree the cress, cucumber, celery juice and ice cubes very finely in a blender on the highest setting. Put in a glass, garnish with the cress and the cucumber slice.

Salsa Mexicana

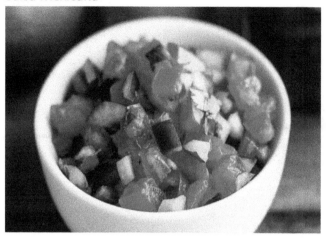

ingredients

- 4 onions
- 3 garlic cloves
- 400 g peeled tomatoes (1 small can; filling weight)
- ½ fret coriander
- ½ fret flat leaf parsley
- salt
- pepper

Preparation steps

1. Cut the peppers lengthways, remove the seeds, wash and chop. Peel and finely chop onions and cloves of garlic. Wash the herbs, shake dry and chop. Bring everything to the boil together with the tomatoes (including the juice) in a saucepan. Season with salt and pepper.

2. Pour the sauce into jars that have been rinsed with hot water, close and allow to cool. Let steep for at least 24 hours before serving.

Tahini and eggplant stew

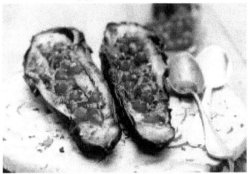

ingredients

- 2 tbsp olive oil
- 1 onion (red)
- 2 cloves of garlic
- 900 g tomatoes
- 1 1/2 tbsp Kotányi VEGGY Classic
- 2 eggplant
- 2 tbsp tahini
- 4 tbsp basil
- 2 tbsp sesame seeds

preparation

1. For the tahini and aubergine stew, first heat olive oil in a large saucepan. Roughly chop the onion and garlic clove and sauté in the oil.
2. Wash and roughly chop tomatoes and add to the saucepan. Add the Kotányi VEGGY Classic and simmer with the lid closed for 20 minutes until the tomatoes have dissolved.
3. Slice the eggplant and add to the tomatoes and continue to simmer with the lid closed until tender.
4. Stir in the tahini, then wash and roughly chop the basil and stir in as well.
5. Season to taste with salt and pepper.

6. Serve tahini and eggplant stew in deep plates and garnish with sesame seeds.

Red smoothie

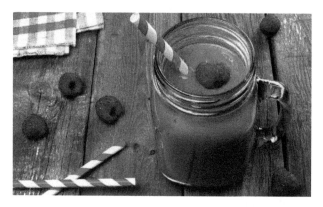

ingredients

- 1/4 pineapple
- 1/2 bunch of parsley
- 1 apple
- 1 cup of raspberries (fresh or frozen)
- 100 ml water (as required)

preparation

1. For the red smoothie, first peel the pineapple and cut into small pieces.
2. Cut the apple and chop the parsley. Put all the ingredients in a stand mixer. Add water as needed. Mix everything well.
3. Pour the red smoothie into a glass and serve.

Orange and carrot smoothie

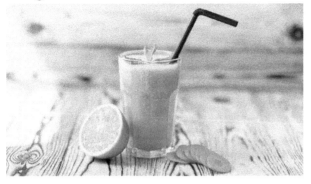

ingredients

- 100 g carrots
- 1 orange
- 1 tbsp sunflower seeds
- 100 ml buttermilk
- 1 tbsp cress

preparation

1. Wash and finely grate the carrots. Peel the orange and cut into large pieces.
2. Put the carrots and oranges together with the sunflower seeds and buttermilk in a blender and puree very finely.
3. Add the cress and serve.

Mango and passion fruit smoothie

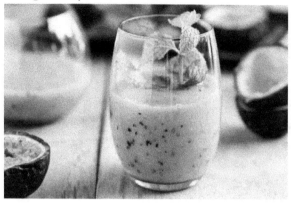

ingredients

- 1 mango (very ripe)
- 2-3 passion fruit
- some mint (or lemon balm, for garnish)

preparation

1. For the mango-passion fruit smoothie, first peel the mango, cut the pulp from the core and roughly chop it. Halve the passion fruit and scrape out the stones with a spoon.

2. Puree the mango and passion fruit in a blender. Fill into glasses and garnish with mint or lemon balm if necessary. Serve the mango and passion fruit smoothie immediately.

Avocado and ginger smoothie

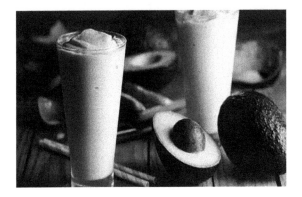

ingredients

- 1 avocado (ripe)
- 1/2 lime (juice)
- 1 apple (green)
- 1 piece of ginger (the size of a thumbnail)
- 1/2 cucumber
- 2 sprig (s) of mint

preparation

1. For the avocado and ginger smoothie, first peel the avocado and remove the core. Mix immediately with the lime juice. Core, peel and roughly cut the apple into pieces and add to the avocado. Peel the ginger and cucumber and add them as well.

2. Mix all ingredients well. If you want, you can add a few ice cubes. The avocado and ginger smoothie garnish with sprigs of mint and serve immediately.

Hearty green smoothie bowl

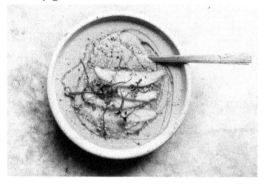

- Preparation:15 minutes
- servings 4

ingredients

- 100 g peas (freshly peeled or frozen)
- 25 g watercress
- 10 g nasturtiums
- 100 g baby spinach
- 10 g herbs (parsley, basil)
- 500 ml vegetable broth
- 2 tbsp olive oil
- 30 g wheatgrass (powder; 3 tbsp)
- 2 tsp lemon juice
- salt
- pepper
- nutmeg
- 40 g dried goji berries (4 tbsp)

Preparation steps

1. Put the peas in boiling water for 5–8 minutes. Then rinse in cold water and let drain.

2. In the meantime, wash water cress, nasturtium, spinach and herbs, shake dry, put some of the two types of cress aside for the garnish; coarsely cut the rest.
3. Finely puree everything with the peas, approx. 300 ml vegetable stock and oil in a blender.
4. Dilute the smoothie with the rest of the broth to the desired consistency. Stir in wheatgrass powder and season everything with lemon juice, salt, pepper and a pinch of freshly grated nutmeg. Divide the smoothie in bowls, sprinkle with the remaining watercress, nasturtium and goji berries.

Colourful vegetable soup with olives

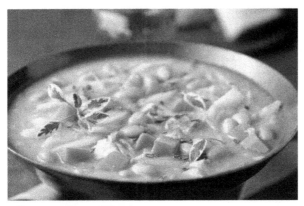

- Preparation: 20 min
- cooking 45 min
- servings 4

ingredients
- 2 carrots
- 1 waxy potato
- 1 pole leek
- 2 poles celery

- 1 tuber fennel
- 2 garlic cloves
- 2 tbsp olive oil
- 1 l vegetable broth
- 2 small sprigs of thyme
- 1 red pepper
- 80 g black olives
- 5 stems herbs z. b. chives, parsley or basil
- salt pepper from the mill
- 1 tsp fruit vinegar

Preparation steps

1. Peel the carrots and potatoes and cut into pieces. Clean and wash the leek and cut into strips. Wash the celery, remove the threads if necessary and cut into pieces about 0.5 cm thick. Clean, wash, halve the fennel, remove the stalk and cut into strips.

2. Put the fennel greens aside. Skin the garlic and dice it. Fry in hot oil in a large saucepan until translucent. Add the leek, potato, carrots, celery and fennel and deglaze with the stock. Put in the thyme and simmer gently for 15–20 minutes.

3. In the meantime, wash the peppers, cut them in half, remove the seeds and white inner skins and dice them. Drain the olives and add to the soup with paprika for another 3 minutes. Then wash the herbs, shake dry, finely chop together with the fennel greens and add both. Season to taste with salt, pepper and vinegar. Serve spread out on plates or bowls.

Pea and mint cakes

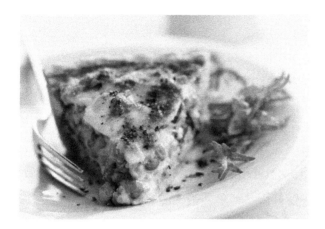

ingredients

- 600 g peas (freshly peeled or frozen)
- iodized salt with fluoride
- 5 g mint (3 stems)
- 50 g sheep cheese (9% fat)
- 60 g whole grain breadcrumbs (4 tbsp)
- 1 egg
- 5 g cornstarch (1 teaspoon)
- pepper
- cayenne pepper
- 10 g chives (0.5 bunch)
- 100 g yogurt (1.5% fat)
- 2 tsp lemon juice
- 200 g salad mix
- 1 cucumber
- 2 tbsp rapeseed oil

Preparation steps

1. Put the peas in boiling salted water for about 5–8 minutes, rinse in cold water and drain well. Puree half of the peas

with a hand blender and place in a bowl; put the other half aside.

2. Wash the mint, shake dry, pull off the leaves and chop finely. Cut the sheep's cheese into small cubes. Add the reserved peas, breadcrumbs, mint, cheese, egg and the starch to the pea puree and stir to form a batter. Season with salt, pepper and cayenne pepper and leave to soak for about 20 minutes.

3. In the meantime, wash the chives, shake dry and cut into rolls. Mix yoghurt with lemon juice and chives to make a dressing and season with salt and pepper. Wash the mixed lettuce and spin dry. Clean and wash the cucumber and cut lengthways into thin slices.

4. Bake the cakes one after the other in a coated pan. To do this, heat 1 tablespoon of oil, add 4–6 small portions of batter and bake for 4–5 minutes on each side over medium heat. Use up the remaining dough with the remaining oil.

5. Arrange the cakes with mixed lettuce and cucumber on plates and drizzle with the dressing.

Curry lentil soup with celery

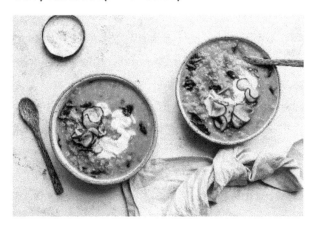

ingredients

- 20 g red lenses
- 200 ml classic vegetable broth
- 1 tsp curry powder
- 25 g celery (0.5 small stick)
- salt
- pepper
- 1 tbsp yogurt (3.5% fat)

Preparation steps

1. Bring the lentils and broth to the boil in a saucepan. Add curry powder and cook covered for 6 minutes over low heat.
2. In the meantime, wash the celery, drain, clean and remove threads if necessary. Put the celery greens aside.
3. Cut the celery into about 5 mm thin slices, add to the lentils and cook covered for another 3–4 minutes.
4. Rinse the celery greens, shake dry and cut into coarse strips.
5. Season the curry lentil soup with salt and pepper. Sprinkle with celery greens and serve with the yogurt.

Healthy vegetable juice with ginger

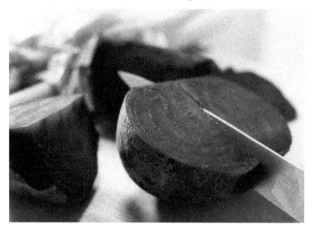

ingredients

- 1 cucumber
- 1 large beetroot
- 5 bars celery
- 2 carrots
- 25 g piece of ginger (1 piece of ginger root)
- 1 tsp argan oil

Preparation steps

1. Wash the cucumber and quarter it lengthways.
2. Wash, clean and quarter the beetroot.
3. Wash, clean and remove the celery from the celery. Wash the carrots and cut off the ends.
4. Wash the ginger and cut into pieces.
5. Process vegetables in the juicer, mix with argan oil and drink immediately.

Spicy carrot cocktail with nasturtiums

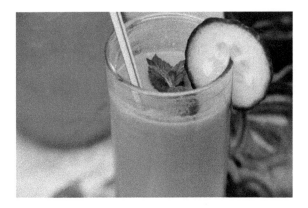

- Cooking time 15 to 30 min
- Servings 4

ingredients

- 20 g nasturtium (with flowers; or watercress; 0.5 bunch)
- 1 clementine
- 100 ml carrot juice (without sugar)

Preparation steps

1. Wash nasturtiums and shake dry well. Put 1-2 beautiful flowers aside, roughly chop the rest of the cress.
2. Halve the clementine and squeeze out. Mix the juice with the cress, carrot juice and ice cubes in a blender. Pour into a glass, pour in mineral water and garnish with capuchin flowers.

Radish and herb cold bowl

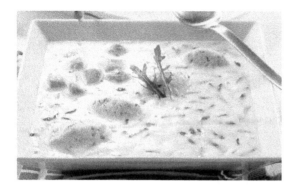

- Cooking time 15 to 30 min
- Servings 2

ingredients

- 250 ml buttermilk
- 3 tbsp lemon juice
- 150 g yogurt (1.5% fat)
- 100 ml milk (1.5% fat)
- 20 g cream of horseradish (1 tbsp; glass)
- salt
- pepper
- nutmeg
- 200 g radishes (1 bunch)
- 40 g mixed herbs (e.g., parsley, mint, basil, chives; 2 bunches)

Preparation steps

1. Mix the buttermilk and lemon juice with the yogurt and milk. Add the horseradish and mix. Season to taste with salt, pepper and freshly grated nutmeg.
2. Wash and clean the radishes and cut or grate into fine sticks. Mix half of the radish rasp into the soup.

3. Divide the soup into 2 bowls. Wash the herbs, shake dry, chop and spread on the soup. Sprinkle with the remaining radishes and season with a pinch of freshly grated nutmeg.

Cold melon and tomato soup

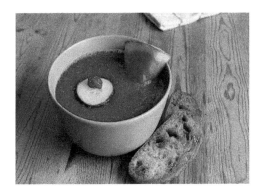

- Preparation: 15 minutes
- cooking time 1 h 15 min

ingredients
- 1 organic lemon
- 1 kg small watermelon (0.5 small watermelons)
- 400 g peeled tomatoes (can; filling quantity)
- sea-salt
- pepper
- 4 stems basil
- 4 tbsp yogurt (3.5% fat)

Preparation steps
1. Wash the lemon with hot water, rub dry and finely grate half of the peel. Halve and squeeze the lemon.

2. Halve the melon with a large knife. Cut into wedges, core, peel and dice. Put the peeled tomatoes and the liquid in a tall container.

3. Add the lemon peel and juice and puree with a hand blender. Salt, pepper and cover and leave to stand in the refrigerator for 1-2 hours. Just before serving, wash the basil, shake it dry and pluck the leaves off. Serve the soup with basil leaves and 1 tablespoon each of yogurt.

Cucumber, apple and banana shake

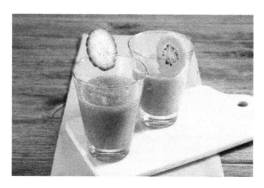

ingredients
- 1 lemon
- 1 banana
- 4 tart apples (e.g., granny smith)
- 1 parsley
- ½ cucumber
- mineral water to fill up
- 10 dice ice cubes

Preparation steps
1. Halve the lemon and squeeze out the juice. Peel and dice the banana. Clean, wash and quarter the apples, remove

the core and dice the pulp. Mix the apples with the banana cubes and lemon juice.

2. Wash parsley, shake dry and chop. Clean and peel the cucumber, halve lengthways, remove the core and cut into bite-sized pieces. Place 3 slices of cucumber on 4 wooden skewers.

3. Finely puree the remaining cucumber pieces with fruit, parsley and ice in a blender. Divide between 4 glasses, fill up with mineral water to the desired consistency and garnish with 1 cucumber skewer each.

cucumber drink with papaya and orange

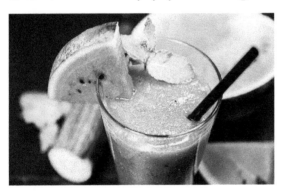

ingredients

- 200 g ripe papaya
- 250 g mini cucumbers
- 250 g oranges
- ice cubes

Preparation steps

1. Peel half papaya, dice the pulp and place in a blender with the seeds.

2. Wash the cucumber thoroughly, cut 2 thin slices and set aside. Peel and dice the rest of the cucumber and put it in the blender as well.

3. Peel the oranges thick enough to remove the white skin. Cut two slices from one orange and set aside.

4. Dice the remaining oranges. Put in the blender with the ice cubes and puree everything on the highest level. Put in a tall glass and garnish with cucumber and orange slices.

Soy and cress mix

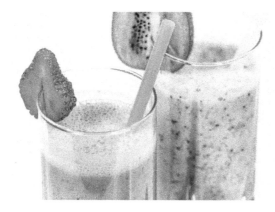

ingredients
- ½ box garden cress
- 250 g cucumber (0.5 cucumber)
- 2 tsp paprika powder (hot pink)
- 100 ml soy drink (soy milk) (1.2% fat)
- salt

Preparation steps
1. Cut the cress from the bed with kitchen scissors and place in a stand mixer or a tall container.
2. Thoroughly wash half the cucumber, rub dry, clean, cut in half, core and dice.

3. Put 1 1/2 teaspoons of paprika on a plate. Moisten a glass on the top with 1 piece of cucumber and press it into the paprika powder to create an even red edge.
4. Puree the cress with cucumber cubes, remaining paprika powder, soy drink, a pinch of salt in a blender, or a hand blender and pour into the prepared glass. Crush the ice cubes in an ice crusher and add carefully.

Chervil shake

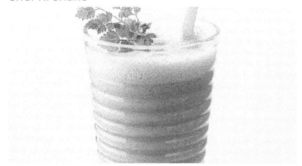

- Preparation:10 min

ingredients
- 2 chervil
- 250 ml celery juice
- 450 ml buttermilk
- salt
- pepper from the mill
- chervil to garnish

Preparation steps
1. Wash the chervil, shake it dry, chop it roughly, mix well with the celery juice in a blender, add the buttermilk, mix up again and season with salt and pepper.
2. Fill into glasses and serve garnished with chervil.

Colourful vegetable soup with white cabbage

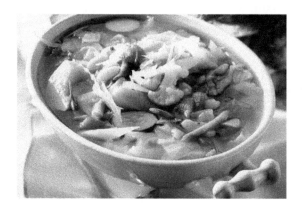

ingredients

- 200 g white cabbage
- 1 zucchini
- 100 g green beans
- 2 tomatoes
- 200 g pumpkin pulp
- 2 carrots
- 2 poles celery
- 1 l vegetable broth
- 100 g cauliflower florets
- 200 g white beans (can)
- salt
- pepper from the mill

Preparation steps

1. Clean and wash the white cabbage and cut into bite-sized pieces. Clean, wash and slice the zucchini. Clean, wash and halve the green beans.

2. Dip tomatoes briefly in boiling water, remove, rinse with cold water and peel off the skin. Cut the pulp into cubes.
3. Dice the pumpkin. Peel the carrots, cut in half lengthways and cut into slices. Clean and wash celery and cut into small pieces.
4. Bring the stock to the boil and add the cauliflower, white cabbage, green and white beans, pumpkin, carrots and celery. Simmer over medium heat for about 5 minutes. Add the zucchini and tomatoes and let simmer for another 3–4 minutes. Vegetables should still have bite. Finally, season with salt and pepper.

Spicy vegetable cocktail

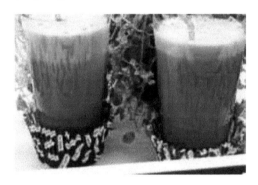

ingredients
- 300 g small green pepper (2 small green peppers)
- 5 spring onions
- 200 g celery (2 sticks)
- 200 g cucumber (1 piece)
- 200 g broccoli
- 12th small tomatoes
- 2 pinches of salt
- green tabasco at will

Preparation steps

1. Halve, core, wash the peppers and cut into large pieces.
2. Clean and wash the spring onions. Clean and wash celery and, if necessary, remove threads.
3. Wash the cucumber piece thoroughly, rub dry and cut into pieces.
4. Trim and wash broccoli and cut into florets. Wash the tomatoes, put 4 tomatoes aside for the garnish.
5. Juice the rest of the tomatoes with bell pepper, spring onions, celery, cucumber and broccoli in a juicer. Season to taste with salt and green Tabasco to taste, pour into glasses with ice cubes and garnish with the tomatoes set aside.

Pineapple buttermilk smoothie

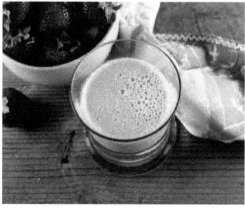

Ingredients

- 1 ripe pineapple
- 6 stems mint
- 500 ml buttermilk (cold)

- 30 g agave syrup (2 tbsp)

Preparation steps

1. Peel the pineapple, cut off the leaves and stem end. Quarter the pineapple, remove the stalk and cut the flesh into small pieces.
2. Wash mint and shake dry. Pluck leaves from 2 stems and finely puree with pineapple, buttermilk and agave syrup in a blender.
3. Fill the smoothie into 6 glasses and garnish with the remaining mint and serve immediately.

CONCLUSION

The detox diet is nothing more than a low-calorie diet, often particularly restrictive, followed by plenty of food for short periods after periods (e.g. anniversaries, holidays) to purify the body from toxic substances accumulated in the previous days. It is a common belief that to detoxify our body, we need liquid meals or smoothies, draining herbal teas and alkaline foods (fruit and vegetables in general). However, there is no scientific evidence that such a practise has any kind of positive health effect.

The body does not require detoxifying foods or supplements that, by the way, do not exist. Our organs, especially the liver, contribute to eliminating metabolic waste and toxic substances, making food detoxification practises completely useless every day.

Certainly, after a period in which you have given yourself a little more in terms of food, especially if you are trying to lose weight or maintain physical shape, a mini-period of greater energy restriction can be a good solution. But there is no reason to eliminate certain foods or follow extreme practises that can do more harm than good, such as prolonged fasting or the consumption of numerous draining herbal teas.

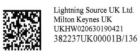

Lightning Source UK Ltd.
Milton Keynes UK
UKHW020630190421
382237UK00001B/136

9 781801 976411